A GUIDE TO
COMPETITIVE VOUCHERS IN HEALTH

A GUIDE TO
COMPETITIVE
VOUCHERS
IN HEALTH

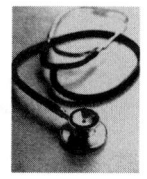

THE WORLD BANK

Library of Congress Cataloging-in-Publications Data

A guide to competitive vouchers in health.
    p. cm.
  Includes bibliographical references and index.
  ISBN 0-8213-5855-3
    1. Medical care, Cost of—United States. 2. Medical care—Finance—United States.
I. World Bank.

RA410.5.G855 2004
338.4′33521′0973—dc22

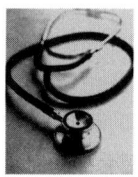

TABLE OF CONTENTS

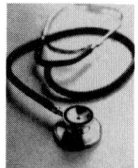

FOREWORD

The *World Development Report 2004* reviews traditional approaches to public service delivery and discusses how they have often failed the poor. Whether in health, education, or infrastructure, supply-side subsidy strategies to fund inputs—such as staff costs, equipment, and buildings used in delivery—have not improved the access to quality services among the poor. An important question remains for developing countries and the international development community on how to deliver and target public subsidies in ways that promote efficiency and innovation, increase accountability for performance, and leverage public resources with private participation and financing.

The output-based aid (OBA) approach seeks to partially answer this question by using a demand-side subsidy delivery strategy. An OBA scheme contracts a private party to deliver services and makes disbursement of the public funding contingent upon actual services delivered. Vouchers are one type of OBA approach. They have the potential to target specific segments of the population effectively, stimulate both supply and demand for under-supplied services, and establish a relatively straightforward monitoring mechanism. When the voucher scheme is built on the principle of competition, it can not only further empower clients by allowing them to bring their business to providers of their choice but also give incentives for service providers to be innovative, cost effective, and responsive to the clients.

Competitive vouchers, however, are one of many types of demand-side subsidy strategies, and only a partial answer to the forthcoming challenges in the health sector. Design and implementation arrangements can affect the effectiveness of the vouchers scheme significantly. This guide aims at providing policymakers and donors with the tools needed to determine the appropriateness of competitive vouchers, as well as information on the design, execution, and monitoring of projects under this type of scheme. We look forward to the use of this guide as a way to facilitate the decisionmaking process regarding alternative options for the delivery of public health services to the poor.

Ellis J. Juan
Manager
Infrastructure Advisory Services
Infrastructure Economics and Finance Department

July 2004

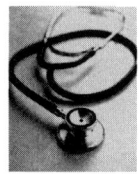

PREFACE

This guide identifies the advantages of competitive voucher schemes in delivering subsidies; describes the circumstances under which they are superior to other subsidy mechanisms; and explains how to design, implement, monitor, and evaluate a voucher scheme. It provides a broad outline of the problems faced by health systems, the rationale for government intervention, and the different ways in which governments and donors subsidize health care.

The guide does not advocate greater use of vouchers but simply raises awareness about voucher schemes, offering policymakers guidance on the choices and decisions they need to make. It also highlights some pitfalls of voucher schemes and describes the different formats vouchers can take depending on the health problems being addressed and the objectives policymakers wish to achieve.

ACKNOWLEDGMENTS

This guide was prepared by a team led by Chiaki Yamamoto and Jeff Ruster. Peter Sandiford, Anna Gorter, Micol Salvetto, and Zil Rojas of Instituto Centroamericano de la Salud (ICAS) prepared the guide. Kathy Khuu and Kwadjo Asante also worked on this guide, and Rosario Bartolome provided invaluable administrative support.

The team greatly benefited from comments and advice from Abdo Yazbeck, as well as participants of the workshop Competitive Vouchers for Health Care Service Delivery held at the World Bank on April 22, 2004. The team is grateful to Ellis Juan, the manager of Infrastructure Advisory Services, and Hossain Razavi, the director of Infrastructure Economics and Finance, for their support and guidance.

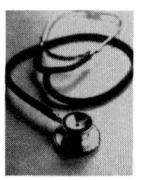

PART I

WHAT ARE
HEALTH CARE VOUCHERS
AND
HOW DO THEY
WORK?

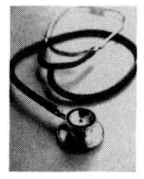

CHAPTER 1

DELIVERING PUBLIC SUBSIDIES IN HEALTH CARE

Health systems in developing countries face enormous problems. In all of the poorest countries—and even in most rich ones—health outcomes vary widely by socioeconomic group. Governments and insurance companies alike are struggling to meet the costs of ever-increasing public expectations for health services. In many countries, households in which a family member suffers from a chronic disease are driven into (or kept in) poverty by the catastrophic cost of ongoing medical care. At the same time, vast sums are being wasted on ineffective—or even harmful—interventions, and enormous technical inefficiencies plague the delivery of health services. Worst of all, there is good evidence that public subsidies in health are failing to reach their main intended beneficiaries—the poor and vulnerable.

WHY DO GOVERNMENT SUBSIDIES DO SO LITTLE TO HELP THE POOR?

Government intervention in the health sector has typically been supply-side subsidies delivered through a network of publicly owned and operated health facilities. Some of these facilities serve the entire population; others cover only those unable to afford health insurance and not covered by social security. In many countries, these services have succeeded in reducing infant and maternal mortality. But few governments in developing countries have raised sufficient revenue to provide the range of services that meets the public's expectations, and government regulations have resulted in serious allocative inefficiencies, with staff often taking precedence over equipment and drugs.

In the poorest countries, the "public" system is really a mixture of publicly funded staff and consumables funded privately through out-of-pocket spending by patients. In many countries, staff also expect informal "fees" in return for access to health care. As a result, the cost-effectiveness of service delivery is low, and services are consumed by relatively well-off patients with less urgent health needs, undermining both the efficiency and equity of the health system.

Supply-side subsidies, which cover some or all of the costs of health services inputs (infrastructure, staff, drugs, equipment, nonmedical consumables), provide little incentive to attract patients or increase productivity. As a result, despite relatively low wages, publicly operated services have remarkably high unit costs, and utilization rates are often low. The absence of targeting (restricting benefits to a certain subset of the population) greatly dilutes the impact of public expenditure on health care. Middle-class people pay less than they can afford, while the poor often pay more.

The perception—and reality—of low quality in the public sector allows the private sector to flourish in developing countries. As a result, many countries see an abundance of private providers, not all of whom provide high-quality services, while the population, particularly the poor, underconsume public services.

WHEN ARE SUBSIDIES FOR HEALTH SERVICES JUSTIFIED?

Three factors make subsidizing health care desirable:

1. *Inequitable distribution of wealth and health.* Society views some redistribution as fair and desirable, particularly to alleviate or eliminate poverty and to give all people the opportunity to enjoy a reasonable standard of health. Health (but not necessarily health care) is generally considered a human right. In the absence of subsidies, as long as the distribution of wealth is inequitable, the distribution of access to health care—and therefore of health status—will also be inequitable. Skewed distributions of wealth and health are not only unfair in their own right, they also create conditions in which catastrophic health care costs can drive some people into poverty or force them to forgo the health care they need. Catastrophic health care costs can be reduced by risk-sharing strategies, such as health insurance and social security, but even in industrial countries the markets for these services operate imperfectly because of asymmetric information. As a result, many people end up falling through the safety net.

2. *Presence of externalities.* Many health interventions—vaccinations, treatment of communicable diseases, removal of vector breeding sites—benefit not only the person being treated but others as well. Family planning is also associated with positive externalities, or spillover effects, since limiting the number of children reduces a variety of social costs associated with excessive population growth.

3. *Incomplete information.* Individuals lack knowledge about their future health care needs and their costs. This uncertainty creates a market for pooling risks and sharing costs through health insurance. Because individuals have some information on their likely future health care costs, however, there is an incentive for those with the highest expected needs to purchase more health insurance than those who expect to have relatively low expenditures. This problem, known as adverse selection, combined with a tendency to overconsume services that are paid for by a third party (a phenomenon known as moral hazard) can lead to complete collapse of the health insurance market or to unaffordable premiums for a large section of the population, exposing them to the risk of catastrophic health expenditures. Subsidies for health education and regulation may help address this source of market failure.

DEMAND-SIDE VERSUS SUPPLY-SIDE SUBSIDIES

Subsidies can be divided into two main groups: supply-side subsidies and demand-side subsidies. Supply-side subsidies are linked to inputs; demand-side subsidies are linked to outputs (figure 1-1). Each type of subsidy has advantages and disadvantages. The two can be used in combination to take advantage of the benefits each has to offer.

Supply-Side Subsidies

Supply-side subsidies cover some or all of the costs of the inputs to health services. They fall into two broad categories: cash subsidies and in-kind subsidies.

Cash subsidies may or may not specify the inputs they subsidize. They include lump-sum payments and block contracts to provide a set of services; tax rebates (on the construction of health facilities in underserved areas, for example); and capitated payments based solely on a catchment population. (A capitation payment that depends on the number of patients actually using a provider regularly or a system in which patients lose access to service when they shift to a different provider is a demand-side subsidy, as it is linked to the output of service utilization.)

The publicly owned and operated national health systems of many countries are examples of in-kind supply-side subsidies. In-kind subsidies are often provided for a more limited range of goods and services, including drugs, donations or loans of premises for health facilities, training, and payment of staff salaries.

Supply-side subsidies are usually relatively simple to introduce and inexpensive to administer, and they can provide benefits to broad population groups. They are appropriate where the subsidized good or service can be used only by the target groups. Examples include immunizations; drugs used to treat communicable diseases, such as tuberculosis, and health facility infrastructure and staff costs in poor areas.

There are several disadvantages to providing supply-side subsidies:

- *Difficulty targeting.* There is no guarantee that supply-side subsidies benefit those for whom they are intended. One way of restricting benefits to target groups is to subsidize the providers they use, but target populations may not use the facilities that receive assistance. Another option is to subsidize inputs that can be used only for specific health

Figure 1-1. Demand-Side Versus Supply-Side Subsidies in Health Care

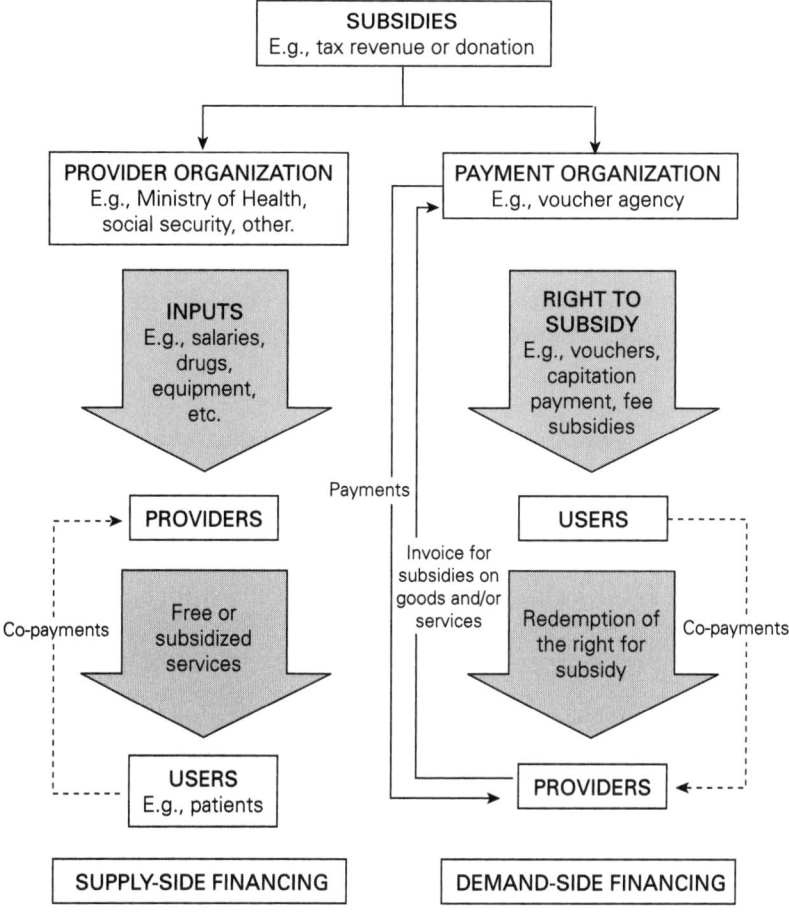

problems, such as immunizations and certain drugs for treating tuber-culosis. The scope of this type of subsidy is limited, however, and may not be sufficient to achieve the desired health system objectives.

- *Lack of patient empowerment.* Supply-side subsidies are often associated with low-quality service. Because assistance flows from the government to the provider rather than to patients, supply-side subsidies create no incentives for service providers to provide good service or offer patients anything beyond the bare essentials in terms of comfort and privacy.

- *Lack of incentives to improve efficiency.* Since supply-side subsidies do not normally link payment to the provision of service, they may be dissipated in salary increases and inefficiency rather than used to improve the quality and increase the quantity of services provided.

Demand-Side Subsidies

The key defining feature of a demand-side subsidy is the direct link between the intended beneficiary, the subsidy, and the desired output (such as access or utilization). The level of funding received by the provider therefore depends on the outputs produced.

Demand-side subsidies can be consumer led or provider led. They can be provided before or after service utilization.

Consumer-Led Demand-Side Subsidies Provided before Service Utilization
Consumer-led demand-side subsidies transferred before service utilization include cash transfers to patients, contributions to or tax rebates on family medical savings schemes, and vouchers. Features of these are:

- Cash transfers provided to potential patients to pay for health care risk being used for other purposes, such as buying food, unless urgent medical care is required.

- Contributions to or tax rebates on family medical savings schemes require families to deposit a certain percentage of their earnings into accounts, which can be used only to pay for medical expenses. (An example is the Medisave program in Singapore.) Making such deposits tax deductible is one way of subsidizing them. Governments can also make deposits on behalf of the poor.

- Vouchers are not always consumer-led demand subsidies (they can also be held by providers). Chapter 2 describes competitive voucher schemes as a form of demand-side subsidies.

Consumer-Led Demand-Side Subsidies Provided after Service Utilization
Cash refunds to patients represent consumer-led demand-side subsidies that are transferred after service utilization. This type of subsidy is commonly used by insurance companies, but it could also be used for public subsidies in a well-developed health system. The major concerns with such a subsidy scheme are the need to ensure that claims for refunds are

legitimate (that is, that service was actually provided) and to avoid moral hazard. The moral hazard problem is reduced if the refund covers only part of the expenses.

Provider-Led Demand-Side Subsidies Provided before Service Provision

Provider-led demand-side subsidies transferred before service provision include cost-per-case contracts in which the provider receives a fixed subsidy for a specified number of services, capitation payments, and referral vouchers distributed by providers that entitle the recipient to goods or services provided by others.

- Cost-per-case contracts are normally channelled by third-party purchasers, such as district or regional health authorities. In a variant of this mechanism, the cost-per-volume contract, a minimum volume of service is purchased, with the cost changing as the volume increases.

- Under capitation a provider receives a subsidy for providing particular individuals with access to care. Capitation payments are demand-side subsidies only if they are tied directly to the number of patients actually served by the provider—as they are in the United Kingdom, where funding follows patients if they change general practitioners. Capitation payments made to providers for covering the residents of a particular zone, irrespective of whether they use a particular provider, are supply-side subsidies. Capitation can be made as payment for providers' own costs and expenses or as payment for providers' purchase of services on behalf of their patients. In the now obsolete British model, general practitioners received a fixed amount of money per patient (weighted by age, gender, and other characteristics), which they used to purchase external services, such as elective surgery, on behalf of their patients.

- Referral vouchers can enable providers such as general practitioners to act as gatekeepers for public subsidies, ensuring that the subsidies are directed to the poorest individuals or those most in need of health care. Limiting the number of vouchers received by each provider can control the total volume of subsidies. Making the number of vouchers received by each provider dependent on the number of target patients reached can create an incentive for careful rationing of these subsidies. Such a system makes it possible for medical professionals to retain some of their discretionary power to consider the merits of individual cases, but allowing them to do so also introduces some risk of abuse.

Provider-Led Demand Subsidies Provided after Service Provision

Provider-led demand subsidies transferred after service provision include fee-for-service subsidy claims and target payments. Under a fee-for-service subsidy, the provider receives a subsidy from the government for having provided eligible services to eligible individuals. An example is the New Zealand General Medical Subsidy, in which general practitioners receive a payment from the government for each child consultation they give. Receipt of the subsidy may be made conditional on the provider limiting or eliminating the fee paid by the patient. This form of provider subsidy may be administratively simpler than a voucher scheme, but it can be more difficult to control, as an independent mechanism is required to verify that the service was actually provided. Fee-for-service subsidies have also been criticized for leading to too little service among subsidized groups. They do provide a strong incentive to increase productivity, as the provider's subsidy income is directly related to the rate at which the services are provided.

Target payments are made to providers who achieve certain predefined service targets. In the United Kingdom, general practitioners receive subsidies conditional upon achieving specified coverage levels for immunization. The subsidy is usually not based on individual patients but on some population target, such as vaccination or screening coverage rates. Subsidies could also be based on a health outcome among a particular population, such as the cure rate for tuberculosis patients. The key to successful target payments is the ability to independently (and cheaply) verify their achievement.

Advantages and Disadvantages of Demand-Side Subsidies

Demand-side subsidies have several advantages:

- *Output-based remuneration.* By tying the receipt of subsidy to the generation of some output, demand-side subsidies create incentives to increase those outputs and therefore raise productivity.

- *Evidence-based practice.* The link between subsidies and outputs creates an opportunity to specify what the outputs will be. This is important for two reasons. First, it enables the subsidies to be used explicitly to address health problems for which a solid justification exists. Second, it allows policymakers to specify interventions that are known to be evidence based and cost effective. Many health care services have little impact on health. They are provided partly because of incomplete information (patients often do not know if an intervention is effective), partly because of moral hazard, and partly because of the agency problem—the fact that patients' ignorance of the impact of health interventions can lead them to allow providers with financial incentives for delivering services to make decisions on their behalf. Demand-side subsidies allow the agency role to be partially assumed by the donor to ensure that patients receive evidence-based, cost-effective care.

- *Targeting.* Targeting can greatly improve the ability to meet the equity and poverty-reduction objectives of subsidies. It can also increase the consumption of services associated with positive externalities. Although targeting can be achieved indirectly with supply-side subsidies, it is possible to directly target individuals only when receipt of the subsidy is linked to provision of the service. Targeted consumer-led demand subsidies, such as vouchers, are one of the few instruments that allow health planners any degree of certainty that their subsidies are reaching the intended population groups. Perhaps more important, vouchers enable health planners to know who has not been reached, provided that good records are kept on who receives the vouchers and who uses them. This form of targeting is particularly valuable when trying to extend services to populations that are difficult to reach (sex workers, drug addicts, indigenous populations). Receiving vouchers intended specifically for them may make these groups feel that the services they receive will cater to their needs. By doing so, they may increase usage. Care must be taken, however, to ensure that targeting does not lead to stigmatization.

- *Output-based monitoring and evaluation.* Monitoring is often thought of as a mundane activity carried out mainly to stop people (including staff) from abusing the system. For traditional supply-side assistance, it often comes down to checking whether or not certain items have been purchased and distributed and whether or not planned activities have been carried out. Monitoring may involve looking at whether the investments are being put to their expected use, but it rarely examines what happens to individuals as a result of assistance. With demand-side subsidies, it is possible to trace exactly who receives services, what services they receive, and even what outcomes are achieved. This information makes it possible to evaluate the system. Being able to identify the fruits of an investment is something that politicians—who must approve subsidies—like very much. The public also likes evaluations, which show tangible benefit from their tax contribution. Demand-side subsidies are not without their drawbacks, however:

- *Higher transactions and administrative costs, because of the need to quantify outputs.* Transactions and administrative costs—including the costs of producing and distributing vouchers, contracting providers and monitoring their performance, reimbursing providers, and establishing systems to avoid abuse of the voucher scheme—can be substantial.

- *Overservicing.* Overservicing can occur because of the direct link between outputs and subsidies, combined with moral hazard and agency problems.

- *Cream-skimming.* Cream-skimming occurs when providers avoid providing care to groups that require more services than others. As under capitation payments and health insurance subsidies, this problem can arise if the subsidy is for providing access to services rather than their utilization.

- *Lower patient satisfaction.* Capitation subsidies create no incentives for providers to make services convenient or comfortable for patients. They can encourage providers to take on more patients than they can adequately handle and to treat them with the bare minimum of consumables.

The greatest disadvantage of demand-side subsidies is probably the higher transaction and administrative costs. The choice between supply-side and demand-side subsidies often therefore boils down to whether or not the expected benefits of higher productivity and quality outweigh the higher overhead costs.

OTHER FACTORS INFLUENCING THE EFFECTIVENESS OF SUBSIDIES

Three other factors—competition, contracting, and corruption—also affect the effectiveness of health care subsidies.

Competition

Subsidies are justified because a free market for health care services fails to address such issues as externalities and the distribution of health benefits across different income groups. Subsidies, however, often create other problems—including problems that are even more serious than those they were intended to solve. The common practice of restricting subsidies to publicly owned and operated facilities impairs competition in the market for health services. This loss of competition alters incentives in a way that often undermines efficiency, quality, and patient satisfaction.

Preserving choice and competition in subsidy schemes has the additional advantage of not leading to, or entrenching, parallel or duplicated health infrastructure. Subsidies make use of existing health services, regardless of who owns them. In the main cities of many developing countries, the government, the social security institute, and the private sector each own separate hospitals and clinics, all serving the same geographic areas. Competition for subsidies makes it possible to contract services from any of these providers, based on which offers the best prices, quality, or both. Competition for subsidies prevents them from distorting the market for health services in the same way that noncompetitive subsidies do. Competitive subsidies do not prevent new providers from establishing services (by unfairly subsidizing others). In fact, by making such investments more profitable, they can encourage the establishment of new facilities in previously underserved areas or the development of new services to address health problems that had been neglected. Demand-side subsidies also do not prevent inefficient providers whom few patients choose from closing down. Finally, demand side subsidies open the public sector, where efficiency and quality are often lowest, up to competition.

Do different types of benefits differ in terms of the benefits they yield? Consider the following scenarios:

- *Subsidies are given in the absence of competition (for example, to a single public sector provider).* This is the benchmark scenario, against which the others are compared. For supply-side subsidies, improving services to attract more patients does not alter the amount of subsidy received. The subsidies therefore create little or no incentive to attract more patients by improving patient satisfaction or lowering prices. For demand-side subsidies, attracting more patients generates a proportionate increase in revenue. In the absence of competition, then, demand-side subsidies provide incentives to attract patients, which supply-side subsidies do not.

- *Subsidies are given to all providers competing in a market.* Under this scenario, patients have a choice of providers, and a level playing field is established. The competitive environment will create incentives to increase efficiency and improve patients' perceptions of quality. There is no financial incentive to improve quality that cannot be perceived by potential patients. Thus, although competition creates an incentive to improve efficiency and patient-perceived quality, supply-side—but not demand-side—subsidies have a tendency to undermine this incentive, particularly if they are large in relation to total provider revenue.

- *Subsidies are given only to accredited providers.* Governments may provide subsidies only to providers who can demonstrate that they meet certain quality standards. This limits choice for patients, but if successful it can ensure that they receive better service. The benefits of including some form of accreditation with subsidies accrue directly and indirectly— directly by ensuring that the subsidized services meet certain standards, indirectly by creating an incentive for providers to raise their service standards to meet the requirements for accreditation. As under the second scenario, supply-side—but not demand-side—subsidies have a tendency to undermine the incentive to improve efficiency and patient-perceived quality, particularly if they are large in relation to total provider revenue.

- *Providers must compete for limited places in a subsidy scheme.* This scenario goes a step beyond accreditation, effectively introducing an additional competitive process. Limiting places in a subsidy scheme limits choice for patients, but in many cases it lowers administrative and monitoring costs. This form of competitive subsidy may be used to avoid duplication in the supply of services that require high initial investments and services for which the number of potential beneficiaries is relatively low. Like accreditation, competition for limited places in a subsidy scheme can be used to improve quality in areas that patients are unable to perceive. It can also drive down costs. With supply-side subsidies, there is probably a stronger incentive to compete for places in the scheme than with demand-side subsidies, because once selected the provider is sure that it will receive the subsidy (with demand-side subsidies, the provider must still compete to attract patients eligible for receiving the subsidy). However, that additional level of competition may be important for maximizing efficiency and patient satisfaction.

Even when patient satisfaction is not closely correlated with technical quality, it may still be worth increasing. If patient satisfaction is low, utilization of services will be low, reducing the ability of a scheme to meet its objectives.

Contracting

Contracting can be hugely beneficial, because it forces each party to a contract to specify its expectations. Contracts thus force health planners to consider precisely which services they want from providers and to identify them through detailed patient management protocols and quality specifications. At the same time, the contracting process forces providers to understand purchasers' priorities. This helps them reconfigure the care they provide based on purchasers' demands. Contracts can be more explicit about desired outputs and quality of care specifications under demand-side subsidies than under supply-side subsidies.

Corruption

Leakage—the loss of program funds to people other than the intended beneficiaries—through corruption and theft occurs under both demand-side and supply-side subsidies, but the form that it takes can be quite different under the two types of schemes. Vouchers are susceptible to counterfeiting and black markets. Fee-for-service and capitation subsidies are vulnerable to submission of fraudulent claims. Supply-side subsidies can be diverted through pilfering, reselling, or using donated inputs (including staff time) for patients other than intended beneficiaries. Many subsidy schemes are susceptible to providers distorting or falsifying the information they send to donors in order to receive larger allocations than they are entitled to.[1]

---

[1] Cross-subsidies—in which some individuals effectively subsidize others, through differential pricing of services, for example—represent a third group of subsidies. They are not considered here.

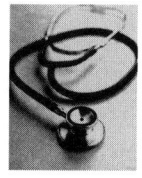

CHAPTER 2

BENEFITS OF COMPETITIVE VOUCHER SCHEMES FOR HEALTH

A voucher is a token that can be used in exchange for a restricted range of goods or services. Vouchers tie the receipt of cash to particular goods, provided by particular vendors, at particular times. Health care vouchers are used in exchange for health services (such as medical consultations or laboratory tests) or health care consumables (such as drugs).

This guide examines voucher schemes as means of subsidizing health care goods and services. It focuses on schemes that involve some form of competition between providers of health goods and services, that provide the bearers of the vouchers with choices, and that involve the private sector. It does not address voucher schemes in which the voucher can be exchanged for cash as an incentive to use health services.

HOW DOES A VOUCHER SCHEME WORK?

A typical competitive voucher scheme works in the way shown in figure 2-1. For voucher schemes distributing public subsidies, the process begins with the transfer of funds to a voucher agency (1). Vouchers are then produced by a voucher agency and distributed to a target population, either by the agency itself (2a) or by third-party organizations (2b), which in turn distribute them to sections of the target population with which they have close links (2c). Voucher recipients take the vouchers to a health service provider of their choice (3) and exchange them for goods or services (or use

Figure 2-1. How Does a Voucher Scheme Work?

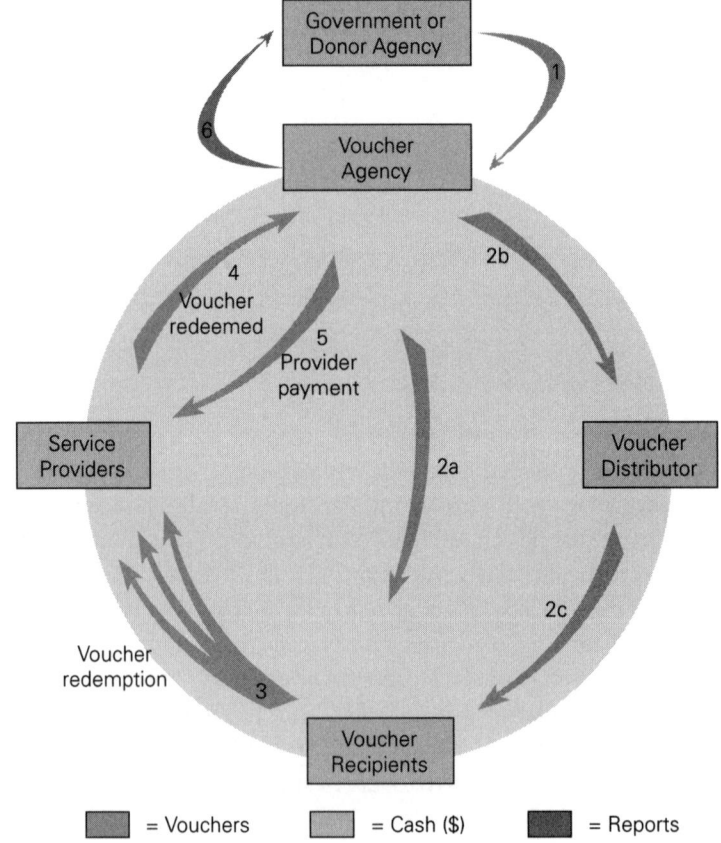

them as partial payment for them).[1] The service providers return the vouchers to the voucher agency (4), along with any other information it requires. The agency then pays the provider a sum, agreed on in advance, for each voucher returned (5). The voucher agency reports the program outputs and outcomes back to the government or donor providing the subsidies (6).

WHAT ARE THE ADVANTAGES OF HEALTH VOUCHERS?

Health vouchers are a specific type of demand-side subsidy. They have certain advantages over other types of demand-side subsidies, but they often entail higher transactions costs. In deciding whether to use a voucher scheme to deliver subsidies, policymakers must determine whether the ability to deliver subsidies more efficiently or effectively outweighs the additional administrative costs. They must also consider some of the limitations of vouchers.

Vouchers Allow Targeting of Beneficiaries

Voucher schemes have greater scope for targeting than other demand-side subsidies. Targeting helps policymakers reach a higher proportion of the people they want to subsidize—a feature known as sensitivity. Targeting also helps exclude people who are not in the target group—a feature known as specificity. In many subsidy schemes, it is often difficult at the level of the health facility to separate those whom one wants to assist from those whom one does not. As a result, sensitivity and specificity are low. Voucher schemes can sometimes improve sensitivity and specificity, because the vouchers can be handed directly to target group individuals in the community, where they can often be more reliably identified. This is particularly true when intended beneficiaries operate outside the law (for example, illicit drug users and, in some countries, commercial sex workers and men who have sex with men) or fear stigmatization (for example, people with tuberculosis, leprosy, and HIV/AIDS). Community targeting is also useful when individuals outside the target population can falsely claim they qualify for benefits (for example, nonpoor who receive exemptions from user charges intended only for the poor).

---

[1] Health service providers include clinics, informal practitioners, hospitals, laboratories or other diagnostic services, pharmacies, community care service providers, health promoters, ambulances or other transport service providers, and vendors of prostheses.

Vouchers Encourage Use of Underconsumed Services

Health vouchers may encourage people to visit providers they might not otherwise have seen. They are particularly useful for subsidizing services that tend to be underconsumed from a social welfare perspective, such as family planning, treatment of infectious diseases, immunizations, mental health care, and maternal and child health services. They are also useful when knowledge of the existence of services is poorly disseminated within the community.

Vouchers Can Be Easy to Administer

The administrative cost of voucher schemes is one of their main drawbacks. However, they can be administered more easily than other demand-side subsidies. Requiring the provider to present a voucher in order to receive the subsidy can prevent irregularities and false claims. If designed well, the voucher can serve as a receipt and a data collection form, as well as a token of exchange.

Vouchers Reduce Provider-Induced Demand

Since they are controlled by the user, vouchers reduce the problems associated with provider-induced demand. And because they are normally used for a clearly defined and limited service at fixed cost, they probably reduce the risk of subsidies being claimed for more expensive conditions than those actually treated. For example, hospitals sometimes claim subsidies based on the patient's diagnostic-related group. Studies have shown, however, that when it is possibile to assign two different diagnostic-related groups to a patient, hospitals tend to use the one with the higher level of subsidy. Voucher schemes largely avoid this phenomenon, known as diagnostic creep.

Vouchers Work Best for Service Packages of Fixed or Predictable Cost

Voucher schemes seem to work best when a fixed value can be assigned to the benefits they provide. This makes it easy to reimburse providers, who are given an agreed-upon amount for each voucher they return to the agency. This type of arrangement is possible when the services provided

---

Box 2-1. Varying the Service Package According to the Needs of the Patient in Nicaragua

In Nicaragua's HIV/AIDS prevention program, treatment of sexually transmitted infections varies according to the diagnosis. The voucher agency specified the management protocol for each infection and provides facilities with the necessary medicines. In special cases, when additional treatment is required, doctors can ask the voucher agency for reimbursement of additional expenses. The same mechanism operates in the adolescent program, which also has standardized management protocols for a range of services, including counselling, family planning, pregnancy testing, a first prenatal check, and treatment of sexually transmitted infections.

Source: Sandiford, Gorter, and Salvetto 2002b.

---

can be specified clearly in advance and each patient receives exactly the same services. It also works when patients receive different services according to independently verifiable conditions, such as the result of a laboratory test (box 2-1). Alternatively, if the proportion of patients receiving different service packages remains constant, then a fixed constant fee (that is, a weighted average of the fees for each cost category) can be used. Problems are likely to arise, however, when the costs to the provider of attending to voucher-bearing patients vary greatly and unpredictably and are impossible to verify independently.

Vouchers Increase Client Satisfaction

In a competitive voucher scheme, the bearer of the voucher can usually choose a provider. If the voucher covers the full cost of the services or if the cost charged by all providers is the same, the bearer will usually base the choice on perceptions about which provider offers the highest-quality, most convenient, and most comfortable service. Providers will raise the quality of their services in order to attract voucher-bearing users.

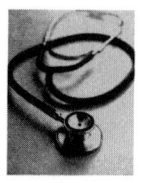

PART II

INTRODUCING
A VOUCHER
SCHEME

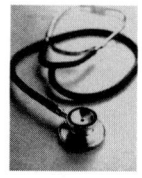

CHAPTER 3

CONDUCTING PREFEASIBILITY STUDIES

Before policymakers can proceed with feasibility studies, they must identify the health sector problem and determine whether public subsidies can help solve it. This stage of the process involves five steps:

- Identify the health sector problem meriting public subsidies and the aims of the voucher scheme.

- Justify the selection of the health sector problem (above others) and the inputs or outputs to be subsidized.

- Identify potential sources of funding.

- Document key stakeholders and their interests, as well as possible partnership opportunities.

- Identify existing service delivery systems that address the problem.

Although each of these stages would appear to follow from the preceding one in a consecutive sequence, in reality neither a voucher scheme, nor any other health program, is always designed and implemented in such a logical process.

IDENTIFYING THE HEALTH SECTOR PROBLEM AND THE AIMS OF THE VOUCHER SCHEME

What problem in the health system are the subsidies going to address? What are the subsidies expected to achieve? Health systems interventions usually attempt to achieve one or more of the following aims:

- Increase the health status of the population.

- Reduce poverty and socioeconomic inequalities in health outcomes.

- Provide services at a lower cost or get more for the same cost.

- Increase patient satisfaction.

Before conducting a feasibility assessment, policymakers should consider which of these (or any other) aims they expect the subsidies will achieve and assign priorities to each. They should also set targets against which to measure the success or failure of the scheme (see chapter 7). Some preliminary data collection might be necessary for a baseline measurement at this stage.

JUSTIFYING THE USE OF A VOUCHER SCHEME

Why are subsidies needed to address the problem? What will the subsidies be used for? Is there evidence that such expenditures are cost effective? Could the subsidies be used more effectively in addressing other health sector problems? Subsidies are justified when the market fails to achieve social goals—a common phenomenon in the health sector. Externalities such as the social costs of high birth rates and communicable disease, socioeconomic inequalities in health, and the risks of catastrophic health care costs are often cited as justifications for subsidies. This is the time to think about whether or not subsidies are really necessary to achieve the aims that have been set. Other forms of government intervention, such as regulation, may be sufficient. Will subsidies introduce other problems? If subsidies can be justified, it is important to write down the basis for this justification before moving on to the feasibility assessment. It is also important to be able to justify the selection of a subsidy scheme over alternatives by demonstrating that it is likely to make a greater contribution to social goals.

If a specific health intervention is proposed, evidence from published international experience that the intervention will yield the expected health outcomes should be cited. Many health sector interventions do not work, and some are even harmful. It is difficult to justify subsidizing interventions that are known to be ineffective (although such interventions are regularly subsidized throughout the world). Much work has been done to separate out and promote evidence-based medical practice.[1] While there will always be a role for innovation and testing of new ideas and strategies, the bulk of health sector interventions should be evidence based.

Figure 3-1 is intended to help guide policymakers in determining whether subsidies are justified and in identifying which type of subsidy is most appropriate to address a given health sector problem.

FUNDING THE SCHEME

There is little point in proceeding to the feasibility assessment stage unless there is at least a reasonable possibility of finding a source of funds to pay for the subsidies. Where will the money for the subsidy come from? Is this source sustainable? The two most likely sources of funding are governments and donors. Existing public funds could also be modified to fund a new subsidy scheme.

---

[1] See the work of the Cochrane Collaboration, available at www.cochrane.org, which prepares, maintains, and promotes the accessibility of systematic reviews of the effects of health care interventions.

Figure 3-1. Decision Tree for Supply-Side Subsidies

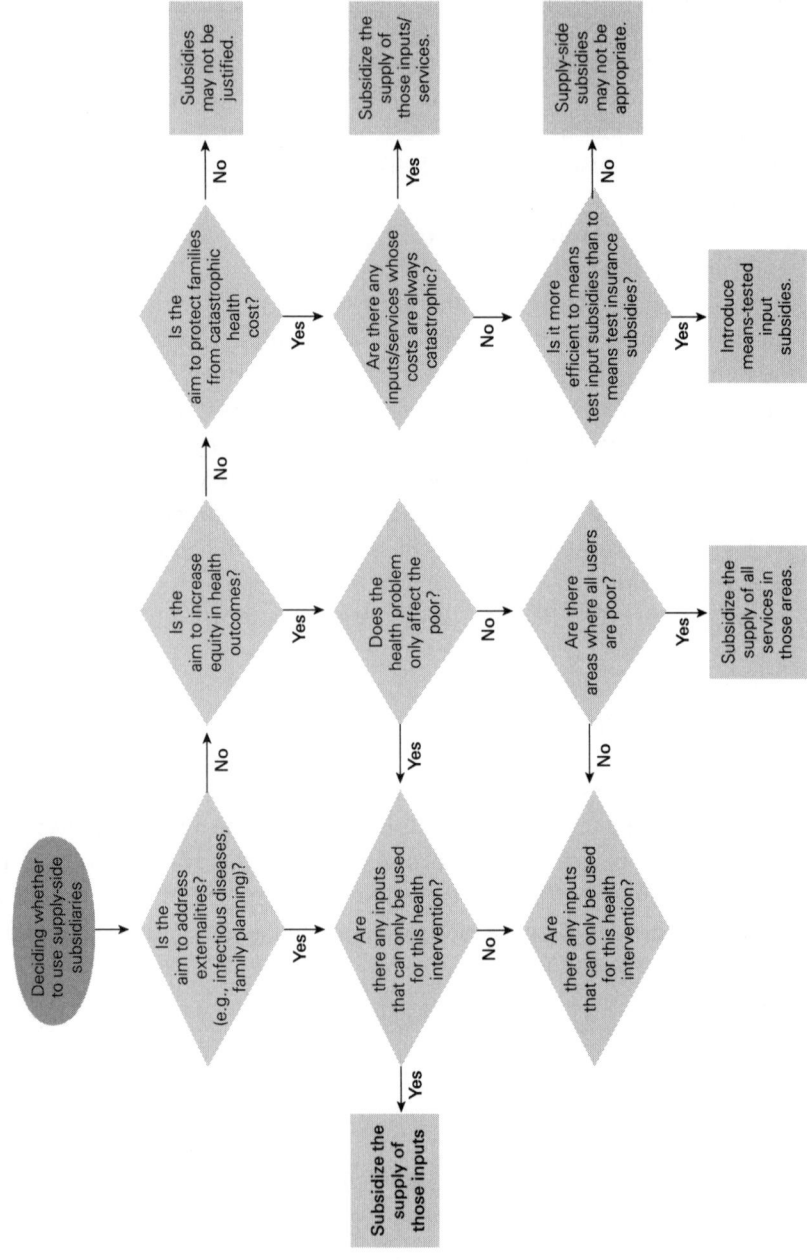

UNDERSTANDING THE CONTEXT IN WHICH SUBSIDIES WILL BE INTRODUCED

Before proceeding to a feasibility study, policymakers need to find out as much as they can about what has been done to address the problem and what opportunities and constraints exist to using a voucher scheme. Some of the questions they need to ask include the following:

- If effective interventions exist, why does the problem persist?
- What is the existing level of service delivery?
- Are services currently being subsidized? How affordable are the services?
- Who are the main stakeholders and what are their interests?
- Who are the intended beneficiaries of the proposed voucher scheme?
- What cultural factors could affect the success of a subsidy scheme?
- What legal and regulatory issues could affect the success of a subsidy scheme?
- What institutional opportunities and constraints exist?

BUILDING PARTNERSHIPS

Who are the likely winners and losers from the proposed subsidies? Can their support for the scheme be achieved? In the process of gathering information on the roles and interests of various stakeholders in the health problem, opportunities may arise to identify potential partnerships and to float the idea of a voucher scheme with potential partners. How open is the ministry of health to a scheme that effectively breaks its provider monopoly over the use of subsidies? How willing would private providers be to entering into a partnership with the public sector, to bid for a contract, to accept vouchers as payment, to sign contracts for services, to follow a strict patient management protocol, to participate in an accreditation scheme? Assessing different stakeholders' reactions can provide a valuable input to the next phase, the feasibility assessment.

Partners may make different types of contributions. Some can provide services, others technical assistance; some can distribute vouchers, others can lobby donors. It is vital to keep an eye out for institutions that could perform the crucial voucher agency role.

Figure 3-2. Decision Tree for Demand-Side Subsidies

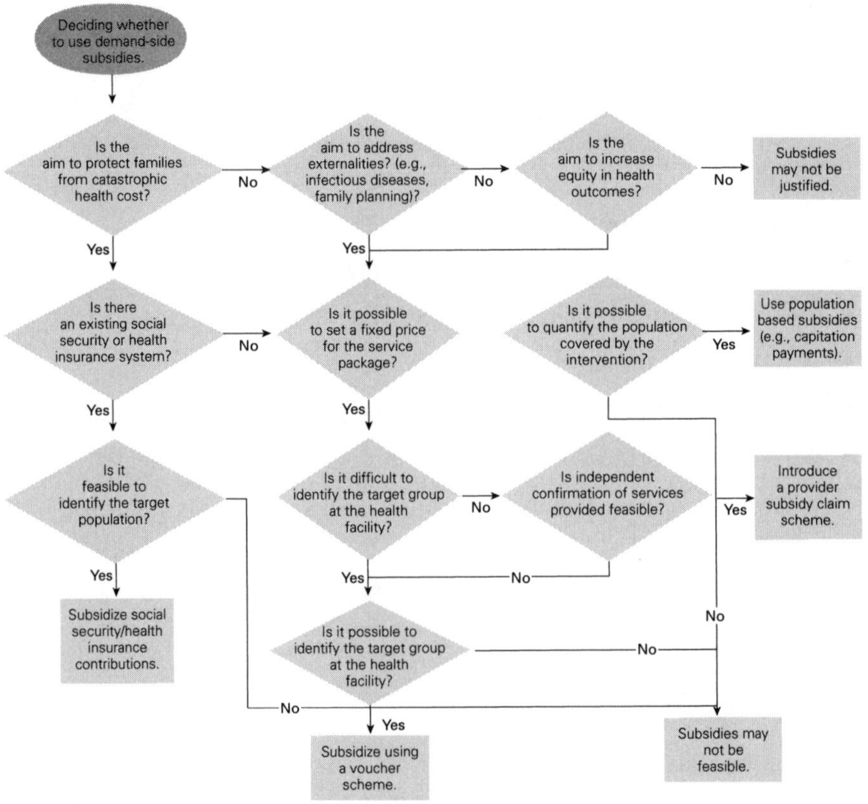

The analysis of existing service delivery may fail to identify some of the potentially most valuable partners. For example, organizations may be working closely with the target population—and therefore potentially valuable partners for voucher distribution—but not currently providing services that address the chosen health problem. These organizations need to be identified at this prefeasibility stage and some idea gained as to their capacity to contribute to the program. Policy makers should keep in mind that partnerships are only tentative at this stage and should be formalized during the design phase when contracts are negotiated and signed.

CHECKLIST FOR FEASIBILITY ASSESSMENT

Before moving on to the next stage in the process, policymakers need to check that they have completed all of the steps in the prefeasibility assessment (table 3-1). An example of such an assessment is shown in box 3-1.

Table 3-1. Checklist for Prefeasibility Assessment

	Yes	No
Has the health sector problem been selected and justified (including target groups)?		
Have sources of potential funding been identified and explored?		
Has the full range of possible interventions been considered and one or more selected on the basis of expected cost-effectiveness?		
Have existing programs and services to address problems been documented?		
Have all other contextual aspects to addressing the problem been recorded?		
Has the full range of possible interventions been considered and one or more selected on the basis of expected cost-effectiveness?		
Have key stakeholders been identified and potential partnerships considered?		

Box 3-1.
Prefeasibility Work on a Voucher Scheme for Cervical Cancer Screening

Problem: Mortality from cervical cancer, the single greatest killer of adult women in Nicaragua.

Aims of voucher scheme: Increase the uptake of screening among poor and high-risk women, improve quality of cervical cytology, ensure follow-up and effective treatment of precancerous lesions.

Justification for choice of problem and use of public subsidies: Externalities associated with social costs of orphaned children if disease is not detected and/or treated on time, socioeconomic inequalities in

continued

Box 3-1. *Continued*

mortality rates, catastrophic health costs of treatment (and some-times even screening), market failure from inability of women to assess quality of cytology. Screening with Pap smear and prompt treatment of precancerous lesions are known to be cost effective.

Potential source of funding: Donors and government; Ministry of Health to provide political support, identify priority areas, pur-chase vouchers and/or request donations, and treat patients with invasive lesions.

Context:

- Poor women and those at high risk of cervical cancer are missed, while younger and better-off women are screened more often than necessary.

- Quality of cervical cytology is poor. No formal training or re-training for cytologists. Inadequate internal and no external quality assurance.

- Inadequate follow-up and treatment, particularly in the public sector. Tendency to overtreat low-grade lesions (possible over-servicing).

- Organization capable of serving as voucher agency exists.

- Good network of public and private sector clinics able to take Pap smears.

- Community health workers and civil society institutions are ca-pable of distributing vouchers and following up with women.

Potential partnerships: The National Cytology Institute can assist in establishing external quality assurance scheme and accreditation system for participating clinics.

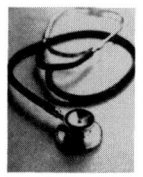

CHAPTER 4

CONDUCTING
A FEASIBILITY
ASSESSMENT

The purpose of the feasibility assessment is to determine whether it is possible to structure the delivery of the proposed subsidies in the form of a voucher scheme. Feasibility assessment also involves making a judgment as to whether doing so is likely to have significant advantages over alternative ways of delivering the subsidies. It may also be necessary to conduct ad hoc studies or pilot tests to determine whether a voucher scheme is feasible and desirable.

The objectives of the feasibility assessment include the following:

- Determine whether the proposed subsidy scheme has characteristics that make voucher schemes difficult to implement.

- Determine whether the proposed subsidy scheme has characteristics that make vouchers a particularly effective delivery strategy.

- Weigh the pros and cons of providing the subsidy with a voucher scheme.

- Decide whether to proceed with the design of a voucher scheme or to use an alternative strategy.

Figure 4-1 illustrates a typical sequence in carrying out the feasibility assessment. The order in which the activities are performed is not critical, however.

IDENTIFYING POTENTIAL IMPEDIMENTS

Several potential impediments stand in the way of implementing a voucher scheme.

Legal or Regulatory Impediments

Some countries prohibit private medical practice. Lack of private doctors would severely constrain a competitive voucher scheme (although it might still be possible to promote competition among public sector providers). Other countries prohibit public sector providers from receiving cash, which limits the use of monetary incentives. In these cases, public providers cannot receive extra payment from outside or private funding sources, which becomes an issue if, for example, a private foundation were trying to fund the subsidies.

Legal requirements can also undermine the flexibility the voucher agency needs to get a scheme up and running. If the scheme is based in a public sector institution, such as the ministry of health, laws and regulations regarding the contracting of staff or externally provided services may be rigid and bureaucratic. The need to obtain signatures from high-level functionaries for minor expenditures may make a voucher scheme untenable.

There may also be regulatory and even legal impediments to evidence-based, cost-effective best practice, which undermine one of the main advantages of demand-side subsidies. Ministries of health frequently have norms for treating health problems—norms that do not always represent evidence-based best practice or the most cost-effective way of addressing a problem. In some cases, the norms may not have kept up with new technologies. Ministerial norms do not always apply to the private sector. Al-

Figure 4-1. Typical Sequencce of Activities in a Feasibility Assessment

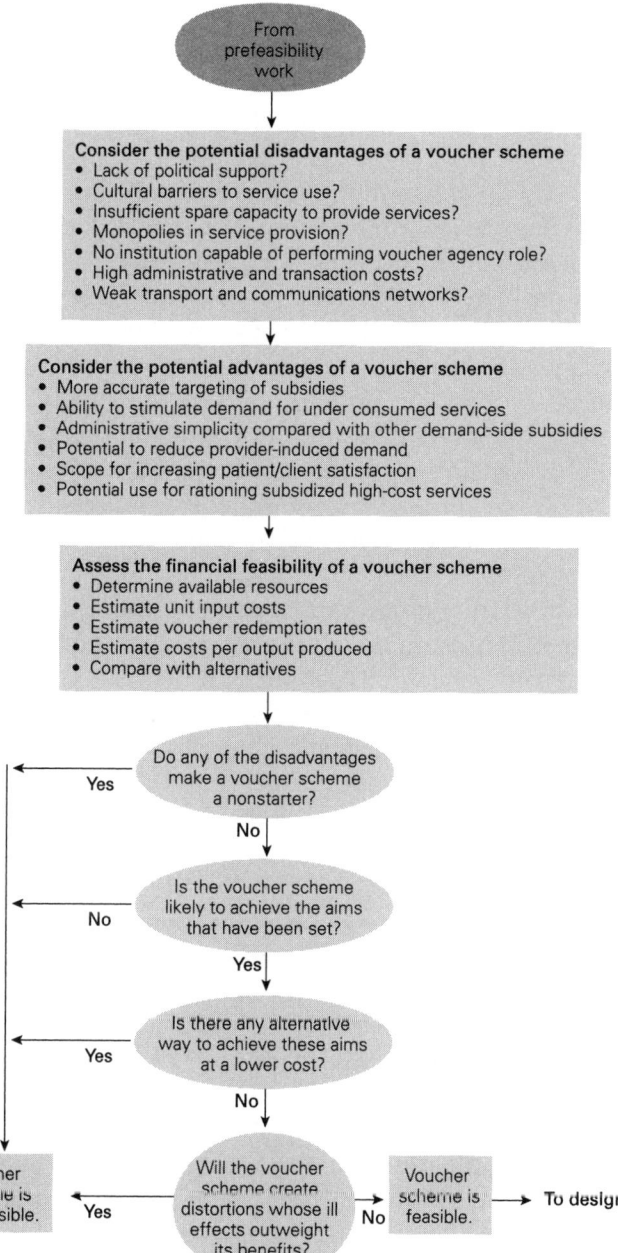

though it may be possible to negotiate exceptions for public sector providers, this should not be assumed in advance.

Lack of Political Support

The importance of political support often depends on the role that the ministry of health plays in the scheme. Even if the voucher scheme is implemented by a private organization or a nongovernmental organization (NGO), the attitude of the ministry of health toward the scheme is likely to be important. For one thing, many donors require the prior agreement of the ministry of health. If government funding is used, the scheme may be introduced and promoted by the ministry of health. Its support may also be required if the voucher will be used at government-owned clinics or hospitals.

Experience has shown that ministry of health officials (and even some donors) often feel that subsidies should be restricted to public sector providers, because they see their role as one of running and improving government hospitals and clinics rather than the broader one of sustaining and improving the health of the population. Government-owned clinics tend to be short of drugs, staff, equipment, and other necessary supplies. It is therefore easy to make a case for prioritizing their rehabilitation before purchasing services from private providers. Ministry of health officials may also view voucher schemes as loosening their control over health sector development funding. Some will probably even have ideological objections to working with the private sector, because they feel that taxpayers' money destined for health care should not end up in private hands. Others may believe that private sector services inevitably cost more than publicly provided services.

Political issues may affect support for the scheme. Voucher schemes can result in poor and underprivileged groups receiving better-quality services than the general population, which can cause resentment. And voucher schemes provide little opportunity for politicians to gain visibility by opening new government-owned facilities. Box 4-1 illustrates what can happen when political factors influence the design and implementation of voucher schemes.

If the ministry of health is to play a significant role in promoting, designing, and running the voucher scheme, other obstacles will also emerge—unless the idea for the voucher scheme is put forward by the highest level of the ministry itself.

Box 4-1.

Political Impediments to Voucher Schemes in El Salvador and Honduras

Political support from the highest level encouraged a donor to support the establishment of a voucher scheme for screening cervical cancer in El Salvador (Calero 2003a). Although it had been made clear that the program was to be run by an independent NGO according to agreed-upon strategies, once the project was ready to be implemented, the technical level at the Ministry of Health expected total control and involvement in running the program. The United Nations agency contracted by the donor to disburse the funding was unwilling to relinquish control, so the Ministry of Health changed the strategy to such an extent that the project became little more than a replication of what the ministry had already been doing in its own screening program. In particular, the ministry restricted the provision of smear-taking services and voucher distribution to its own network of facilities and imposed its own management protocol for patients with abnormal smears—against the expert advice of the project's consultants. The ministry's actions raised the costs of the voucher scheme and diminished the opportunity to prevent deaths.

In a donor-sponsored voucher scheme designed for the prevention of HIV/AIDS in Honduras, failure to secure political support from the outset meant that although funding was secured, the project was eventually abandoned in favor of a traditional supply-side subsidy approach.

Source: Instituto Centroamericano de la Salud.

Voucher schemes for health are virtually unheard of in most countries. Legitimate concerns about potential abuses of the scheme (black markets, collusion between service providers and distributors, counterfeiting) can take on exaggerated proportions. Experience in setting up voucher schemes in diverse settings suggests that it is probably better to begin with small schemes and gradually win support within the ministry of health for expansion, once all of the "teething" problems have been addressed and the program is running effectively. Once officials can see that a scheme leads to improved services for poor and vulnerable groups and that competition between the public and private sector can benefit both, it becomes easier to win support for program expansion.

Sociocultural Barriers to Service Use

The mere distribution of vouchers may not provide recipients with sufficient incentive to overcome sociocultural barriers to using a service. Efforts to encourage vasectomy in men, for example, may be thwarted by a misperception that the intervention leads to impotence. Combining the voucher scheme with social marketing or an information, education, and communication campaign may help remove these barriers.

For some health problems, vouchers may be stigmatizing (box 4-2). People may be reluctant to redeem vouchers—for abortions, emergency contraception, treatment of sexually transmitted infection or tuberculosis—because of the social stigma associated with these conditions and services. In such cases, it is important that the scheme make discretion and respect for patients' confidentiality as priority. Publicity campaigns in the mass media may be counterproductive; alternative ways of promoting the scheme to target groups should be employed.

Lack of Capacity to Provide Services

If service providers are working at full capacity, they will have little incentive to participate in a voucher scheme unless they are paid more than they currently are. With ambulatory care services, there is usually spare capacity or the ability to increase capacity at relatively low cost (by employing another doctor or working longer hours, for example). Capacity limitations are most likely to be encountered for secondary and tertiary care services, such as those requiring the use of operating theaters. These constraints may prove critical. Capacity problems may also be important for services provided by only a few trained specialists; procedures for which there is a lack of inputs (for example, organ transplants); and procedures for which the equipment required is costly and already fully utilized (for example, magnetic resonance imaging).

Box 4-2.
Are Vouchers Stigmatizing?

One of the concerns about Nicaragua's voucher program for the prevention of HIV infection and the treatment of other sexually transmitted infections in sex workers and their clients was that the stigma associated with these vouchers might discourage beneficiaries from keeping and using the voucher (for fear of being discovered by a relative, for example) (Sandiford, Gorter, and Salvetto 2002b). Although this remains a concern, so far it seems that the benefits patients perceive they are receiving from using the voucher are greater than the stigma associated with being singled out as a sex worker or client. Since the scheme began in 1995, care has been taken to avoid publicizing the program, for fear that doing so might increase stigmatization.

In a patient-led partner referral program for control of sexually transmitted infections in the Central African Republic (Koumans and others 2003), vouchers were offered to infected patients to give to their (often asymptomatic) partners for treatment. Although one might have expected some reluctance among patients to refer their partners, well over 90 percent of patients accepted the referral vouchers and 40–50 percent of program participants successfully referred at least one partner.

Lack of a Competitive or Contestable Market for the Services Provided

A voucher scheme does not require competition, but competition can greatly help improve patient satisfaction and productivity. A competitive market is one in which goods or services are produced or sold by a number of different providers. Even in markets with many sellers, perfect competition may not exist. Collusion can allow sellers to fix prices.

Lack of Institutional Capacity to Perform the Voucher Agency Role

The key to a successful voucher scheme depends to a great extent on the abilities and transparency of the voucher agency. To avoid any conflict of interest, the voucher agency should not be part of an organization that provides the services subsidized by the vouchers. It must have the remit, skills, and capacity to negotiate and contract health service providers. Above all, it must be an organization that can be relied on to act honestly and transparently. The voucher agency can be from the public or the private sector (profit-making or nonprofit), and there can be more than one voucher agency for a scheme (more than one agency is often necessary in large countries). A critical criterion is that the agency has the capacity to perform its role and to do so honestly. Financial transparency can be ensured by regular audits, but it is equally important that the organization is—and is perceived to be—objective in negotiating and awarding contracts.

Administrative and Transaction Costs

Voucher schemes can be administratively onerous compared with traditional supply-side subsidies, and there are significant transaction costs associated with negotiating and monitoring contracts. A detailed discussion of this topic appears in chapter 5.

Lack of Adequate Transport and Communications

Voucher schemes require transport and communications networks developed enough to ensure the reliable distribution of vouchers and the timely exchange of information between the voucher agency and other organizations involved. A detailed discussion appears in chapter 5.

IDENTIFYING THE POTENTIAL ADVANTAGES

Voucher schemes are potentially superior to other subsidy delivery strategies because they can more accurately target beneficiaries, stimulate demand for underconsumed services, reduce provider-induced demand, increase patient satisfaction, and ration high-cost services. They are also easier to administer than other demand-side subsidies (see chapter 2).

In addition to these advantages of voucher schemes, policymakers should also consider the advantages of demand-side subsidies generally, if the alternative to the voucher scheme would be a traditional supply-side subsidy. These advantages include the fact that remuneration is based on productivity; that subsidies can be restricted to evidence-based, cost-effective services; that output-based monitoring and evaluation is possible; and that the incentives to improve productivity and client satisfaction are greater for demand-side subsidies than for supply-side subsidies.

DETERMINING WHETHER A VOUCHER SCHEME IS FINANCIALLY FEASIBLE

In the prefeasibility phase, potential sources of funding are identified and explored. In the feasibility phase, policymakers assess whether sufficient resources are available to cover the costs of the voucher scheme, achieve its aims, and do so at a lower cost than alternative subsidy delivery strategies. Costing a voucher scheme can be difficult without having implemented it, but it should be possible to at least draw up a budget. The costs can be divided broadly into the redemption value of the vouchers; those for the voucher agency itself; and those for the logistics required to run the scheme, including marketing, distribution costs, training, production of the vouchers, information system development and maintenance, and external audit.

A major source of uncertainty in costing a voucher scheme is the proportion of recipients who redeem their vouchers. If too few recipients use their vouchers, the resulting health or other benefits may be smaller than expected. Furthermore, the lower the redemption rate, the higher the distribution costs in relation to the outputs achieved. The best way to estimate the likely redemption rate is to perform a pilot test (see chapter 6).

WEIGHING THE POTENTIAL BENEFITS AND OBSTACLES OF A VOUCHER SYSTEM

Ultimately, weighing the benefits of a voucher system and obstacles to implementation become a matter of judgment. It may be helpful to structure this process by answering the following questions:

- Are any of the impediments great enough that they make it impossible to implement the voucher scheme?

- Is the voucher scheme likely to achieve its aims?

- Is there an alternative way to achieve these aims at a lower cost (or to a greater extent for the same cost)?

- Will the voucher scheme introduce distortions into the health system whose effects might outweigh the benefits of achieving these aims?

Box 4-3 illustrates how a feasibility assessment might be conducted for a tuberculosis voucher scheme in the private sector.

CHECKLIST FOR FEASIBILITY ASSESSMENT

Before moving on to the next stage in the process, policymakers need to check that they have completed all of the steps in the feasibility assessment (table 4-1).

Table 4-1. Checklist for Feasibility Assessment

	Yes	No
Have all the potential obstacles, disadvantages, and potential benefits of implementing a voucher scheme been considered?		
Is there a need to conduct any additional studies or pilot tests to reduce areas of uncertainty about the feasibility of a voucher scheme?		
Has a judgment been made as to the feasibility of a voucher scheme?		

Box 4-3.
Assessing the Feasibility of a Tuberculosis Voucher Scheme for Private Practitioners

Prompt detection and treatment of tuberculosis yields positive externalities, in the form of higher economic productivity of the infected person and the preservation of the health of people who otherwise would have been infected. Because tuberculosis disproportionately infects the poor, treatment subsidies also increase income equity in health outcomes. Since the costs of treatment are high, subsidies can also prevent patients from being driven into poverty.

What are the potential benefit and obstacles of using a voucher scheme to treat tuberculosis?

Potential benefits	*Potential obstacles*
• Vouchers can target tuberculosis patients who are difficult to reach.	• Doctors may be reluctant to join a scheme that limits their ability to use nonstandard diagnostic tests and treatment protocols.
• Vouchers offer potential for greater privacy and higher quality of diagnosis and treatment.	
• Demand-side subsidies give private practitioners greater incentive to test and treat tuberculosis. Vouchers simplify the administration of these subsidies.	• National tuberculosis program staff may believe that only public sector clinics should manage tuberculosis patients.
• Demand-side subsidies allow standardized, evidence-based, best-practice management protocols to be enforced in the private sector.	• Many private practitioners are traditional healers, who would not be appropriate for treating tuberculosis patients.
• Providing vouchers for tuberculosis drugs (rather than the drugs themselves) reduces wastage from expired stocks.	• Costs are difficult to estimate in advance.
• Vouchers for diagnostic testing create a strong incentive for laboratories to increase screening of patients.	
• A voucher scheme facilitates information exchange between private practitioners and national tuberculosis control programs.	

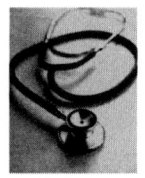

CHAPTER 5

DESIGNING A VOUCHER SCHEME

A voucher scheme can be described in terms of five key policy areas:

- Recipient policies (who is eligible to receive or use the voucher)
- Benefit policies (what services can be paid for with the voucher)
- Price policies (how much the recipient pays to use the voucher)
- Provider policies (which providers can participate in the voucher scheme)
- Value policies (how much the provider receives for each voucher).

The aims of the voucher scheme are specified and prioritized during the prefeasibility phase. In the design phase, a set of policies that is consistent with the stated aims is determined. The various options available are described, and guidelines on which are suitable for achieving different aims are provided.

CHOOSING A VOUCHER AGENCY

Choosing the right voucher agency can make the difference between success and failure. The voucher agency is responsible for producing the vouchers, negotiating contracts with service providers, and reimbursing service providers on presentation of vouchers. It is also usually responsible for monitoring the quality of the services or goods provided. In addition, the agency may be in charge of distributing the vouchers, although it may subcontract or delegate this role to one or several other organizations. If the distribution of vouchers is carried out by other organizations, the voucher agency is usually responsible for identifying these organizations, negotiating with them, and paying for their services if they charge for them.

In choosing a voucher agency, policymakers should place more emphasis on competence and ability to deliver than on political or academic credentials. Furthermore, there need not be just one voucher agency. Indeed, in large countries, it may not be practical to have a single agency, unless the organization has branches nationwide. Another alternative would be to subcontract out the voucher agency role, with different entities working in different areas. Time-limited contracts could be awarded through competitive tender, making the markets for the agencies' services contestable, if not fully competitive. Box 5-1 provides examples of the different types of institutions that have served as voucher agencies.

The voucher agency can be a public sector institution, a private sector institution, or a parastatal organization, which has more independence and autonomy than traditional government departments. Whichever type of institution is chosen, the voucher agency must have four attributes:

- *The voucher agency must be neutral.* It should not have links to any potential service providers, as such links could create conflict of interest. Thus, if ministry of health clinics are participating in the scheme as providers, it may not be appropriate for the ministry of health to serve as the voucher agency. Other public sector institutions, such as the ministry of finance, could be sufficiently independent of service providers.

Box 5-1.
Who Runs the Voucher Program?

Many of the reports on using vouchers in health care fail to document the institutional arrangements for the voucher agency role. But the information that is available suggests that a wide range of alternatives appear to have been used. The Local Initiatives Program in Kolchata, India, was implemented by the Child in Need Institute, a child health and nutrition non-governmental organization. The Nyeri Youth Health Project in Kenya is run by the Family Planning Association of Kenya. The Taiwan (China) coupon scheme for intrauterine devices was administered by the Maternal and Child Health Association, which subsequently became the Planned Parenthood Federation affiliate. In Zambia, an emergency contraception scheme was set up primarily as a research project and run by the University Teaching Hospital (Skibiak, Chambeshi-Moyo, and Ahmed 2001). Ministries of health have also operated voucher schemes. In Indonesia, the Safe Motherhood project, which made the services of private midwives affordable for poor women, was run by the district health authority.

- *The voucher agency must have a good reputation.* The agency is responsible for ensuring the transparency and accountability of the scheme and preventing abuse or misuse of vouchers. Opportunities may arise for collusion between the voucher agency and service providers. External audits may not be sufficient to ensure transparency. In theory, public organizations are more accountable to voters and taxpayers, but they may be just as susceptible to corruption as private agencies. Whichever type of agency is chosen, it makes sense to publish the criteria used for selecting providers and the agreements on fee rates (if they are not established by benchmarks).

- *The voucher agency must have the appropriate range of skills and experience.* Needed skills include the ability to negotiate and contract with service providers and the ability to monitor performance of those contracts, including any quality specifications they may stipulate. General accounting and administrative skills are also required. In most cases the agency will also need skills in the specific area of health being tackled. This raises a problem, as the organizations with these skills tend to be service providers themselves or those with ties to service providers. Such skills can be brought into an organization relatively easily. Similarly, if the voucher scheme is providing services to a particular target population, such as commercial sex workers or people with disabilities, the agency should be familiar with beneficiaries' problems and needs. Some skills can be developed within institutions through training (see chapter 6).

- *The voucher agency must have sufficient autonomy to be able to handle financial management and contract providers.* This is unlikely to be a problem in private organizations, but regulations for government agencies are often strict. Sometimes these regulations can be circumvented by creating parastatal organizations with wider powers.

ESTABLISHING RECIPIENT POLICIES

Recipient policies clearly define the target beneficiaries, the geographic limits of the scheme, or both. Generally, policymakers define the target groups, while the voucher agency works out the operational definitions of eligibility. In an HIV/AIDS prevention scheme, for example, the government could contract with an organization that works with high-risk populations, which would distribute the vouchers to all of its clients. Figure 5-1 shows a decision tree for designing recipient policies.

Establishing Criteria for Voucher Eligibility

Inclusion criteria that can be used in determining the recipient policies include age; occupation (for example, miners, commercial sex workers, migrant workers); location; exposure to specific disease risk factors (for example, smoking, family history, contact with infected carriers); income; ethnic group; disease or health status (for example, tuberculosis patients, pregnant women); gender; sexual orientation; and previous health service usage.

How do policymakers decide who should be eligible for vouchers? Target beneficiaries need to correspond to the aims of the subsidy scheme (table 5-1).

Figure 5-1. Designing Recipient Policies

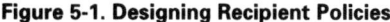

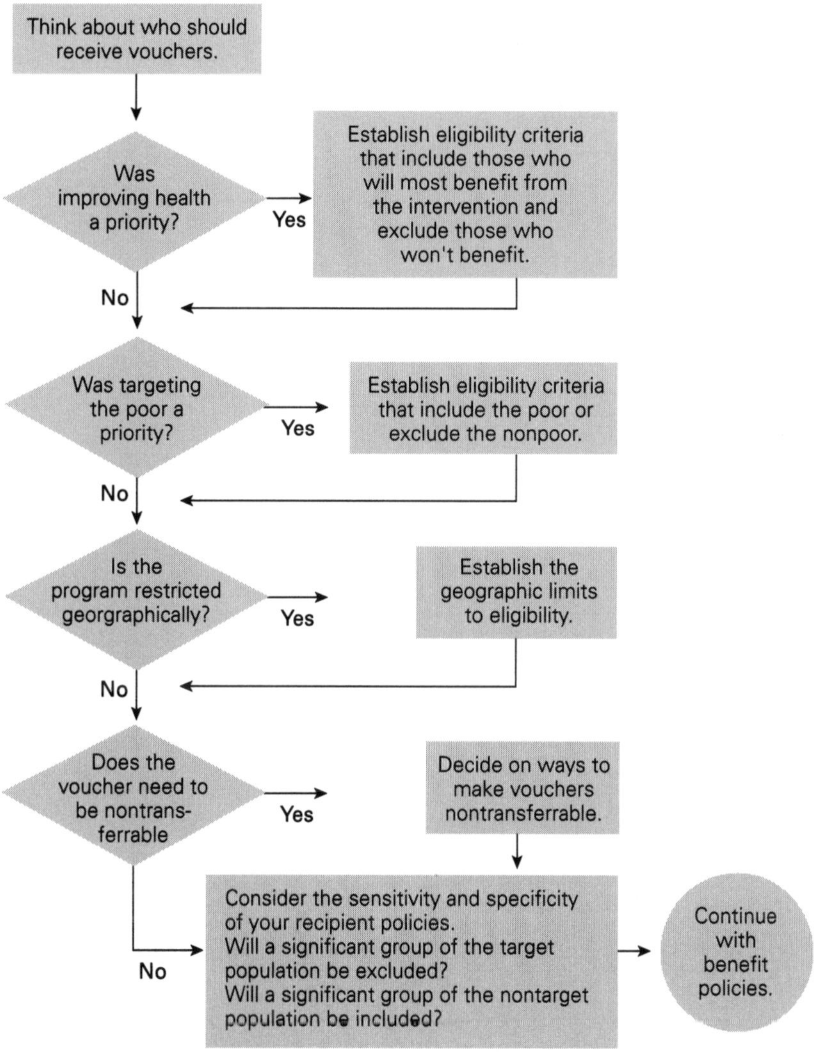

Think about who should
receive vouchers.

Was improving health a priority?

→ Yes → Establish eligibility criteria that include those who will most benefit from the intervention and exclude those who won't benefit.

No ↓

Was targeting the poor a priority?

→ Yes → Establish eligibility criteria that include the poor or exclude the nonpoor.

No ↓

Is the program restricted georgraphically?

→ Yes → Establish the geographic limits to eligibility.

No ↓

Does the voucher need to be nontransferrable

→ Yes → Decide on ways to make vouchers nontransferrable.

No →

Consider the sensitivity and specificity of your recipient policies.
Will a significant group of the target population be excluded?
Will a significant group of the nontarget population be included?

→ Continue with benefit policies.

A program that seeks to increase equity and reduce poverty, for example, should target recipients who are poor. Geographic targeting is one of the simplest ways to reach the poor, but doing so risks including some people who are not poor, but who reside in poor areas, and excluding some poor people who do not reside in poor areas. It also excludes some

Table 5-1. Matching Beneficiaries with Program Aims

Program aim	Target beneficiaries	Country	Reference
Prevent HIV/AIDS by preventing and treating sexually transmitted infections	Sex workers, their partners, and their clients; men who have sex with men; adolescent glue sniffers	Nicaragua	Sandiford, Gorter, and Salvetto (2002b)
Increase use of sexual and reproductive health services among adolescents	All poor adolescents 12–20 years of age in selected regions	Nicaragua	Sandiford, Gorter, and Salvetto (2002b)
Increase screening and treatment of women with preinvasive cervical abnormalities	All poor women 30–59 years of age from villages or provinces in areas selected for their high levels of poverty	El Salvador / Nicaragua	Calero (2003a) / Sandiford, Gorter, and Salvetto (2002b)
Increase use of village midwives by the poor	Poor women who are pregnant or have a child less than one year old	Indonesia	Knowles (2000)
Increase access to emergency contraception among adolescents	Young women in need of emergency contraception	Zambia	Skibiak, Chambeshi-Moyo, and Ahmed (2001)
Increase use of reproductive and child health services in slum areas	All female residents and children of selected urban slums	India	Mookherji (2003)
Reduce child mortality from malaria	All pregnant women who receive prenatal health services	Tanzania / Uganda	Marchant and others (2002) / Root (2003)
Reduce incidence of sexually transmitted infections	Partners of patients with sexually transmitted diseases	Central African Republic	Koumans and others (2003)

of the poorest people, who may not have an identifiable home at all. Other ways to identify the poor, such as means testing, can be more accurate, but they are more costly. Another alternative is to delegate responsibility for identifying the poor to such groups as nonprofit organizations, community health workers, and faith-based organizations that work with impoverished groups. This strategy allows policymakers to increase the accuracy of targeting by varying the number of vouchers distributed to each organization (or even to individuals within the organizations) based on poverty indicators recorded at the time the vouchers are redeemed.

For example, a policymaker gives agency A and agency B 100 vouchers each to distribute among their respective recipient group. Each time someone uses a voucher, his or her income level is recorded. Assume that the groups distribute all 100 and everyone who received a voucher used it. After the first round, the record shows that 80 percent of the voucher redeemers who received vouchers from Agency A are poor, but only 20 percent are poor among those who received vouchers from Agency B. This means that only 100 out of 200 voucher recipients were poor. The next time, the policymaker gives 150 vouchers to Agency A and 50 to Agency B. This time, 130 out of 200 voucher recipients will be poor.

Tradeoffs between Sensitivity and Specificity

Sensitivity—reaching a higher proportion of specific groups—can be increased only at the cost of reduced specificity. Policymakers thus need to decide which is more important, not missing potential beneficiaries or excluding people who do not belong to the target group. In a program intended to provide vouchers to the poor, excluding some poor people may seem unfair. Moreover, if too many poor people are excluded, the impact of the program will be limited. But including too many of the nonpoor wastes scarce program resources and subjects the program to criticism. Policies can be fine tuned to improve the targeting of a program, but improving sensitivity and specificity is costly.

Transferability of Vouchers

Vouchers can be transferable (that is, redeemable by someone other than the original recipient) or nontransferable. The initial temptation is always to make them nontransferable, in order to prevent people other than the original recipients from receiving the benefits of the voucher. But making vouchers nontransferable may be costly. To prevent voucher transfer, one needs to identify the original recipient and have the service provider confirm his or her identity. This can be done in several ways (box 5-2), but they add administrative complexity and cost to the scheme. Policymakers need to consider whether the cost is worth the increase in specificity.

Even if it is possible to prevent people other than the voucher recipient from using the voucher, it may not always make sense to do so. The indirect recipient may well be as poor as the original recipient; where vouchers are targeted according to health need rather than income, indirect voucher bearers may even be in greater need of the service than the original recipients. Furthermore, if one assumes that a high proportion of the direct recipients who give their vouchers to indirect recipients would not have used them, transfer of vouchers may help keep redemption rates high, thereby raising the efficiency of the scheme at producing its outputs.

An alternative to making vouchers nontransferable is to monitor the frequency of their use by indirect recipients and examine the proportion of these recipients that falls into the target group. Doing so provides information upon which to base a subsequent decision to enforce transferability or not. At the end of a consultation, service providers could simply ask bearers whether their voucher was given to them by a friend or a voucher distributor and whether or not they had to pay for it. Collecting this information makes it possible to model the effect of voucher transferability on sensitivity and specificity. If the proportion of indirect recipients becomes too high, or if a black market develops, the possibility of making the voucher nontransferable could be considered.

Policymakers need to ensure that the original recipients are fully aware of the benefits and do not pass on their vouchers simply because they perceive them to be of no value. This is something that should be monitored closely through studies of nonredeemers. Voucher distributors can play a key role in ensuring that recipients are well informed. Their efforts can be reinforced by a clear, well-targeted information, education, and communication campaign.

In some cases, ensuring that vouchers are not transferred is important. Some vouchers entitle the bearer to an expensive service, and considerable effort has been put into identifying suitable recipients. Restricting transfer is particularly important if the goods or services received have a marketable value. This is most likely to be the case where the benefits of the vouchers can be used for diagnosing or treating illnesses other than those

Box 5-2.
How Can Vouchers Be Made Nontransferable?

There are a number of ways to make vouchers nontransferable. Here are a few:

- Write the recipient's name on the voucher and ask the provider to confirm it by asking to see a photo identification card. To ensure that the provider checks the recipient's identification, the provider can be required to fill in the number of the identification card, which the voucher agency can check against a register kept at the time the voucher is distributed. This process may be costly, and many poor people may not have personal identification.

- Have the recipient sign the voucher at the time it is distributed and again when it is redeemed. If a high proportion of the population cannot write, a thumb print can be used instead. The provider can compare the signatures or thumb prints to ensure that they belong to the same person. This is a relatively low-cost technique, but it may make the voucher less attractive to recipients (whether it does so could be checked in a pilot test). Providers may need to be trained to read and compare thumb prints.

- Attach a photograph to the voucher. Photos are expensive, but if the redemption value of the voucher is high, this measure may be justified. This method does not prevent providers from accepting vouchers from people other than those whose photograph is on the voucher, but few voucher bearers will try to use a voucher that carries a photo other than their own. The honesty of the provider can be monitored periodically by the use of "mystery patients" (people with vouchers carrying photos of someone else).

- Take digital images and send them electronically to providers. Digital photos are far cheaper to produce than printed photos.

continued

> **Box 5-2. *Continued***
>
> They can also be sent electronically. A digital photo could be taken at the time the voucher is distributed and sent to the provider by e-mail or posted to a secure Web site. For additional certainty, providers could be asked to make a digital image of the patient, which could be compared with the original. The obvious limitation of this method is the need for digital cameras and universal Internet access by providers. For some target groups, such as commercial sex workers or men who have sex with men, this method may be unacceptable.

the scheme is focusing on (for example, broad-spectrum antibiotics). Nontransferability is more important when the aim of the voucher scheme is to increase equity in health than when the aim is to control communicable disease, since the success of the scheme can be undermined if the voucher is sold to someone better off than the original recipient. Preventing the transfer of vouchers is also important when a core group for the spread of an infectious disease (such as commercial sex workers) is being targeted, since, assuming that the original recipient would otherwise have redeemed the voucher, transferring it to someone not in the core group undermines the scheme's effectiveness in controlling the disease.

DETERMINING BENEFIT POLICIES

Benefit policies define what the voucher entitles its bearer to receive. The benefit can be a specific health service or a package of services. Table 5-2 illustrates the wide range of health services that have been provided through voucher schemes.

Benefit policies are particularly important if health gain/effectiveness is a key objective of the voucher scheme. Benefit policies allow policymakers to define a package of services or a patient management protocol that is derived from evidence-based, cost-effective best practice. The more effective the services covered by the benefit policy, the greater the health gain produced by the scheme. The process of determining the benefit policy

Table 5-2. Benefit Policies of Selected Voucher Schemes for Health

Aim	Benefit	Location	Reference
Provide female contraception through insertion of intrauterine devices (IUDs)	Insertion of IUDs	Taiwan (China)	Cernada and Chow (1970)
Improve family planning and pre- and postnatal maternal health services through village midwives	Package of maternal health care and family planning services	Indonesia	World Bank (2000)
Prevent sexually transmitted infections and HIV, and treat sexually transmitted infections among sex workers and other vulnerable groups	Package of sexual health services, including voluntary counseling and HIV testing	Nicaragua	Gorter (2003)
Improve the uptake and quality of sexual and reproductive health care for adolescents	Package of services, including counseling, family planning, pregnancy tests, prenatal care, and treatment of sexually transmitted infections	Nicaragua	Gorter (2003)
Increase access to and improve quality of cervical cancer screening for poor women	Package of services including screening and treatment for precancerous lesions	Nicaragua / El Salvador	Sandiford, Gorter, and Salvetto (2002a) Calero (2003a)
Provide young people with access to sexual and reproductive health care	Package including diagnosis of sexually transmitted infections, male circumcision, and family planning services	Kenya	Erulkar (2003)
Provide girls with access to emergency contraception through a variety of suppliers	Dose of emergency contraceptive pill	Zambia	Skibiak, Chambeshi-Moyo, and Ahmed (2001)
Provide residents of urban slums with reproductive and child health services	Package of reproductive and child health services	India	Mookherji (2003)

may therefore involve a search of the literature or the employment of a technical expert. Ideally, one should draw up a detailed patient management protocol, perhaps in the form of a flowchart, that covers every conceivable contingency. If management depends on clinical diagnoses or the outcome of laboratory tests, this should be reflected in the protocol.

The benefit policy must be clear to both the voucher bearer and the service provider. If bearers do not know what is excluded, they may have false expectations, especially if a copayment is required (see box 5-3). If providers do not know what is included and excluded, they will not be able to price their services accurately during the tendering process. It is important to specify whether the voucher entitles the bearer only to diagnosis of a disease or to treatment as well. When treatment is included, it should be clear what the treatment is and at what point in the disease process the patient is entitled to it. If, for example, operations for invasive tumors or antiretroviral treatment for people with HIV are excluded, it must be clear. It is customary to print the benefit policies on the voucher itself. If there is insufficient space on the voucher, it may be more practical to print the policies on an accompanying flyer or packaging. It is also important to accurately describe the benefit policies in any social marketing or information, education, and communication campaigns that accompany the voucher scheme.

In most situations, it is wise to establish an expiration date for the vouchers. Setting an expiration date helps limit the financial risks assumed by the voucher agency (which could otherwise be liable for payments after the scheme had officially ended), and it can ensure that the contract with the provider remains in force. Expiration dates also encourage recipients to use the vouchers. Without expiration dates, or with long validity periods, recipients may be tempted to save their vouchers. During this time, they may lose or forget about the vouchers. Having an expiration date also helps in the process of evaluating the uptake strategy. If a short validity period is set, the voucher agency has to be confident that the vouchers can be distributed with plenty of time in which recipients can use them.

DETERMINING PRICE POLICIES

The price refers to what the voucher bearer pays to the provider at the time the voucher is redeemed. This amount can range from nothing, for a fully

---

Box 5-3.
Benefit Policies: The Importance of Stating the Limits

The cervical cancer program in Nicaragua offers a package of services exclusively for screening and treating precancerous lesions.
Although the scope of the benefits was clearly specified both on
the voucher itself and during the social marketing campaign,
some women expected and requested a full gynecological consultation and breast screening. Had the limits of service provision
not been clearly stated on the voucher, this confusion may have
led to serious problems and bad publicity for the scheme.

---

subsidized scheme, to the cost of the services (see box 5-4).[1] The price policy can take the form of a percentage discount off the normal price or a
fixed monetary discount (for example, a discount of $5 off the consulta-
tion price). The price paid by the voucher bearer can be variable, with different discounts given to different groups. Thus very poor people may pay
nothing for services, while others pay 50 percent.

Price policies are particularly important where the main aim of the
voucher scheme is to increase equity or reduce poverty. In these cases, the
voucher bearer must be fully subsidized or pay a price that is well below
the market price. Together with the recipient policy, the price policy determines how effective the scheme will be in achieving its equity and poverty reduction aims.

Price policies can also affect the efficiency of the scheme. Costs that can
be recovered from patients will lower the total cost of the scheme to the
donor or government (or enable it to cover a larger population). But costs
borne by the voucher bearer, no matter how nominal, will deter some
people from using their vouchers. Asking voucher recipients to bear some
of the cost also introduces administrative costs that fully subsidized
schemes do not face.

---

[1] In some voucher schemes, the bearer is paid for using the voucher. These schemes, which
have been used in drug rehabilitation programs, are not considered here.

DETERMINING PROVIDER POLICIES

Provider policies determine who can provide the benefits of the vouchers and under what conditions. They are important for three of the main aims of subsidy schemes, for different reasons. For health gain, provider policies make it possible to select providers with the highest technical quality and therefore the greatest effectiveness of treatment. For technical efficiency, the policies affect how much the scheme costs. For patient satisfaction, a free provider participation strategy can be used that allows patients to decide whom to see.

Box 5-4.
Price Policies Used by Different Voucher Schemes

Voucher schemes can take different approaches to prices.

Box Table 5-1. Price Policies of Voucher Schemes

Program	Location	Reference	Price policy
Female contraception program	Taiwan (China)	Cernada and Chow (1969)	50 percent discount on the cost of inserting intrauterine device
National Insecticide-impregnated Bednet program	Uganda	Root (2003)	Discount of the equivalent of $1 for purchase of net
Randomized trial for mammography screening for women with Medicare	United States		Total exemption from fee or reimbursement of 80 percent of subsidized fee, provided patient meets Medicare deductible
Safe motherhood program (vouchers subsidize services provided by village midwives)	Indonesia	Knowles (2000)	Village midwives can charge only supplemental fees for consumables purchased on open market, such as drugs

La Clínica, the voucher agency and provider of some services in a voucher scheme for migrant farm workers in Wisconsin, has a fixed third-party provider reimbursement schedule (box table 5-2).

continued

Box 5-4. *Continued*

Box Table 5-2. Fees Charged by La Clínica (1992)

Service	Fee
Outpatient care	
Office visit	$15 maximum
Prescription	$5 maximum
Laboratory services	$15 maximum
Dental visit	$35 maximum
Emergency room visit	75 percent of total cost
X ray	75 percent of total cost per X ray
X ray interpretation	75 percent of total cost per X ray
Inpatient care	
Hospital charges	60 percent of charges per admission, up to $500 maximum
Physician charges	50 percent of charges per admission, up to $250 maximum
One-day surgical procedures	
Hospital charges	60 percent of charges per admission, up to $400 maximum
Physician charges	50 percent of charges per admission, up to $200 maximum

Source: Slesinger and Ofstead (1996).

The most liberal provider policy allows any provider to participate in the voucher scheme. Such a policy can be a good idea when it is important to make the services as widely available as possible and when the administrative costs associated with each provider can be kept low. The downsides of a liberal provider policy are that administrative costs are to some extent proportionate to the number of participating clinics and that such a policy does little to control the technical quality of service provided (see figure 5-2).

If the number of providers is restricted, the process of selection should be transparent, so that as many providers as possible take part in the selection process.

Criteria for Selecting Providers

A number of criteria can be used to select clinics for participation in the scheme. The first is cost. Providers can be asked to bid; those offering the lowest bids can be selected. Alternatively, a benchmark price can be established, and clinics offering to provide services to a larger population at that price can be selected.

Figure 5-2. Designing Provider Policies

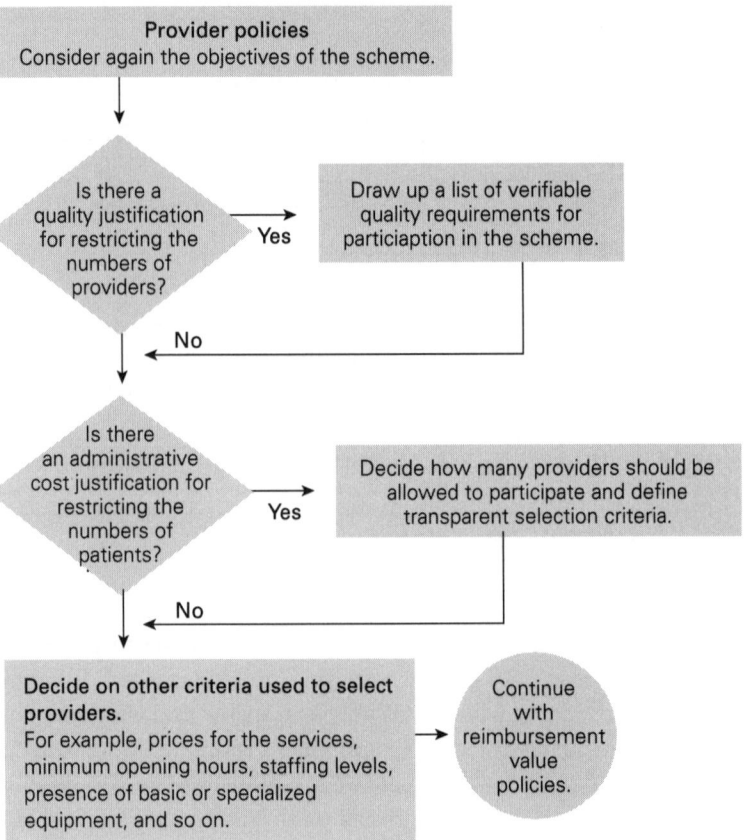

A second criterion for selecting providers is quality. All participating clinics can be required to meet certain minimum standards, including the following:

- Minimum opening hours

- Staffing levels (for doctors, nurses, receptionists)

- Basic or specialized equipment

- Communications, such as e-mail

- Registration with the ministry of health

- Willingness and ability to send samples to laboratories and patient records to the voucher agency

- Performance of staff in proficiency tests

- Average patient waiting times

- Patient satisfaction indices

Some illustrative examples can be found in box 5-5.

Encouraging Providers to Participate

It may be necessary to spend time with providers to convince them of the benefits of participating in the voucher scheme. Where voucher schemes are new, providers may be reluctant to participate. They may wonder whether they will actually be reimbursed for the vouchers they return. Some may find the contracting or accreditation processes intrusive or threatening. Others may object to the loss of autonomy brought about by the imposition of a fixed patient management protocol, details of which they may not agree with. Providers are also sometimes worried that the socioeconomic profile of voucher-bearing patients may undermine the image of their clinics as places attended by the wealthy.

It is difficult to allay all of these fears until providers see the scheme operating in practice. Once the program is operating successfully, some providers who originally refused to participate may express interest in doing so. The scheme needs to create opportunities for such providers to participate.

Box 5-5.
Choosing Service Providers that Meet Program Needs

The cervical cancer screening program in El Salvador needed to contract with a laboratory to provide cytology results, but none of the laboratories tested passed the voucher agency's proficiency test. The lack of a provider encouraged a few professionals who were skilled at reading Pap smears to form a laboratory, which was subsequently contracted by the voucher agency.

In the Zambian emergency contraception voucher scheme, all public maternal and child health units had to be excluded from the list of service providers because of their restricted working hours (Monday to Friday only). Since, to be effective, emergency contraception needs to be taken within 72 hours of unprotected sex, any outlet that could potentially be contracted had to be open 24 hours a day, 7 days a week. The agency eventually chose private pharmacies and hospital outpatient departments. Pharmacies have the additional advantage of anonymity, which is particularly well suited to a sensitive issue such as emergency contraception.

DETERMINING REIMBURSEMENT VALUE POLICIES

The value of the voucher is the amount the provider receives upon returning the voucher to the voucher agency. The simplest mechanism is one in which providers agree in advance to a fixed value for the voucher and all providers receive the same amount. This method is used if a benchmark price is used to select providers.

An alternative is to use the providers' actual tendered price and pay different providers differently. This policy should be pursued with caution, as it can lead to accusations of lack of transparency.

Even more sophisticated policies, which generate incentives for providers, are possible. Payments can be made to voucher distributors based on the number of target group patients treated, on the redemption rate they achieve with their vouchers, or on the socioeconomic profile of patients treated.

In many situations, the service package received by the patient varies, based on clinical diagnoses, laboratory tests, or other reasons. If this is the case, it is important to independently establish verifiable criteria for values that are above the minimum in order to prevent what has been called "diagnostic creep" (the tendency for providers to select higher-value packages). One way to do so is to maintain separate contracts for providers of laboratory diagnostic services or services that merit higher reimbursement values.

Value policies can affect effectiveness of a voucher scheme if they are used as incentives for providing additional services (if, for example, extra payments are made for referring patients for voluntary counseling and testing for HIV).

DESIGNING THE VOUCHERS AND OTHER MATERIALS

Once overall design of the voucher scheme is decided, the voucher itself needs to be designed to maximize the redemption rate of the voucher.

Creating an Attractive Graphic Design

The appearance of the voucher often has an important effect on whether or not the recipient uses it. The voucher should be attractive to recipients and give the appearance that it represents something of value. A modest investment in the services of a graphic designer can pay off handsomely. If the voucher scheme is promoted through social marketing, it is sensible to use the same slogans or images on the voucher as on the promotional material.

Preventing Counterfeiting

A wide range of measures can be taken to prevent counterfeiting. These measures vary in cost as well as the degree of security they confer. Policymakers must assess the risk of counterfeiting and weigh it against the cost of different security measures. Low-cost measures that can be employed to prevent counterfeiting include the following:

- Individually number the vouchers (including check digits).

- Use watermarks.

- Use several fonts.

- Use colored ink stamps.

- Use bar codes for numbering.

- Use self-adhesive seals

- Laminate the vouchers or package them in cellophane.

Of these measures, the first is perhaps the most important, since it enables one to quickly identify duplicate vouchers or vouchers with numbers that have not yet been distributed. Check digits are a more sophisticated measure, based on making one digit of the voucher number the result of a mathematical function of some or all of the other digits. A computer program can quickly detect counterfeit numbers by performing a check as the number is introduced, but this can add to printing costs, since the numbers will not be a simple sequence. Most of the other measures simply add to the cost of producing counterfeit vouchers. Unless counterfeiters think they can easily recover this cost, they are unlikely to make the investment.

Expiration Date

If the vouchers are valid only for a limited time, it is important that the expiration date be immediately visible, especially if the vouchers are in a closed package. If the vouchers come in a closed package, it may be useful for voucher distributors to ask recipients to open the packet upon receipt.

Multiple-Section Vouchers

Sometimes it can help to create a voucher with multiple tear-off or cut-off sections, in which one part of the voucher remains with the bearer, while other parts are returned to the voucher agency or sent to a laboratory with the specimens (box 5-6). It can also be useful to leave a space in the voucher for the patient's signature, to ensure that patients actually receive the health service they were supposed to have received. This signature can be compared with one obtained at the time the voucher is distributed. Doing so can help monitor transfer of vouchers to indirect recipients and detect fraud by providers.

Printing

Because unit printing costs drop dramatically as the number of vouchers printed increases, it is usually worth producing a large number of vouchers at a time, enough for several rounds of distribution. Doing so, however, makes it difficult to change policies. Distributing the voucher with a cheaply produced insert that explains the voucher policies in detail, in particular the benefit policies, allows the policies to be changed after the voucher is printed. It also allows the voucher itself to be small and portable.

Box 5-6.
Designing the Voucher

GinecoBONO, the voucher used in the cervical cancer program in Nicaragua, is sequentially numbered, with the expiration date stamped on top and the services offered clearly stated both inside and outside the packaging, which is a packet or booklet. One part of the voucher, which includes a space to write the appointment for the second visit (to collect test results), is retained by the patient. The other part of the voucher is retained by the clinic. The patient is asked to sign this part of the voucher, which is then returned to the voucher agency as proof that service was rendered.

In the Taiwan (China) female contraception program, the voucher consisted of three detachable parts, each of which served a different purpose. The first part remained with the field worker as a record of distribution, the second and third parts were given to the patient, who handed them over to the physician. The physician held on to the third part as a proof of services delivered. He or she sent the second part by registered mail to the county nurse, who forwarded it to the voucher agency. This part of the vouchers was used for reimbursement of services as well as evaluation and monitoring purposes.

TRANSPORT AND COMMUNICATIONS

Voucher schemes require reliable communications—between the voucher agency and voucher distributors and between the voucher agency and service providers. The voucher agency needs to be able to distribute the vouchers. Providers need to be able to return them, along with any information required, to the voucher agency. Patients sometimes need to be transported to specialist care providers. The logistics involved in organizing reliable transport and communications can be complex (box 5-7). To ensure that they work properly, they should be pilot tested.

If providers are required to send samples to a central laboratory, systems to transport the samples need to be established, along with reliable ways to ensure that providers, patients, and usually the voucher agency receive the results. Producing double (or triple) copies of the results can help.

DISTRIBUTING THE VOUCHERS

Vouchers can be distributed by the voucher agency, by an external agency contracted by the voucher agency, or by providers. In most cases, vouchers can be handed directly to beneficiaries. It is also possible to make the vouchers available at various dispensing points (such as municipalities), where beneficiaries pick them up. This strategy can significantly lower costs. Box 5-8 describes a scheme in which community leaders were responsible for voucher distribution.

Whoever distributes the vouchers, they must reach the intended beneficiaries. If providers distribute the vouchers, beneficiaries will be restricted to those who visit their clinics, and providers may be tempted to give them to patients other than those for whom they are intended, especially if recipient characteristics are not monitored (see chapter 7).

It is important to keep track of whom the vouchers have been given to. The voucher agency should record the serial numbers of the vouchers given to distributors. These simple measures facilitate evaluation of the efficacy of the voucher distribution strategy. They also provide a check on counterfeiting and prevent distribution of vouchers at the point of service delivery.

Box 5-7.
Facing the Challenges of Transport and Communications

Transport logistics can be complex—especially in a region in which some of the areas served are accessible only by plane or boat in the wet season, as is the case in Nicaragua's cervical cancer program. That program has four transport systems in place:

- Health promoters from the voucher agency and private clinic nurses distribute the vouchers. Service providers organize and pay for distribution, which is coordinated and supervised by the voucher agency.

- Medical records, Pap smears, and laboratory results are sent to the voucher agency in the capital by planes, buses, a courier service, and some of the clinics' own vehicles. The cost is shared by service providers and the voucher agency (on behalf of the subsidy provider).

- Community health workers follow up on patients with high-grade lesions who fail to return to the clinic for their results. The workers visit the women and advise them that they need treatment. If this fails, a promoter from the voucher agency is sent. If necessary, the health promoter provides the woman with the money required for transport to the clinic.

- The voucher agency (on behalf of the subsidy provider) pays the expenses of women requiring specialist treatment in the capital if they cannot afford the bus ticket or overnight accommodation.

PAYMENT OF SERVICE PROVIDERS

In the simplest cases, service providers bring or mail in the vouchers and the voucher agency calculates the amount owed, writes a check, has the provider sign a receipt, and records the numbers of the vouchers that have been returned. If a computerized information system is in place, it is not difficult to have it automatically generate receipts for each provider, with

---

Box 5-8.
Using Village Leaders to Distribute Vouchers

Village leaders may be better able to identify the poor than outside agencies, and they can make qualitative judgments that can be more valid than quantitative indicators. Village leaders may be inclined to identify their relatives, friends, and political supporters as beneficiaries, however (Gwatkin 2000). To avoid this, formal methods for identifying the poor that involve village leaders can be used. One such method is the participatory wealth ranking, which uses a community's own definitions and perceptions of poverty and employs rigorous cross-checking methods to ensure consistency and accuracy of results (Simanowitz, Nkuna, and Kasim 2000).

A safe motherhood program in Indonesia has experimented with using village leaders to identify the poor and distribute vouchers to them (Knowles 2000). Under the program, women are eligible if their family eats two or fewer meals per day, their husband has lost his job, some children in the family are not attending school for economic reasons, or the community health center is too far away to be easily accessed from the village. Whether the program has succeeded in targeting beneficiaries remains to be seen.

---

the numbers of the vouchers recorded on them. A decision has to be made as to how often providers are paid for their services. This is a compromise between the wishes of the providers (who like to be paid as soon and as frequently as possible) and those of the agency, for which frequent payment adds to administrative costs.

DEVELOPING INFORMATION SYSTEMS

Design and development of the information system is best carried out once all other design aspects of the scheme have been worked out and the information needs have become clear. Voucher schemes need only information that contributes to decisionmaking or determines actions. There is no point in collecting or recording information that will never be used. The development of information systems for voucher schemes is facilitated by the fact that each voucher represents a self-contained unit, which can be recorded as a single "case" in a computer database.

Data Collection Forms

One of the first steps in designing the information system is designing the data collection forms. Some of the forms and registers that may be used include the following:

- *Registry of voucher distributors (individuals, organizations, or both).* The register should record the serial numbers of the vouchers given to each distributor. The register will help maintain control over voucher distribution and utilization.

- *Registry of voucher recipients.* For each voucher, it is useful to record the date and place of distribution. It can also be useful to obtain the name, address, date of birth, and signature of the recipient in order to monitor transfer of vouchers and to facilitate studies of nonredeeming voucher recipients.

- *Registry of service providers.* Keeping a registry of service providers facilitates both quality control and reimbursement. The registry should include the dates the providers began participating in the program.

- *Clinical and diagnostic records.* Clinical and diagnostic test records can have an important impact on public health policy and planning.

- *Registry of patients requiring follow-up.* It is important to track patients carefully to minimize loss to follow-up. If feedback can be obtained once treatment is complete, it should be recorded.

- *Record linkage.* Ideally, all registries and records should be linked in a common database. It can be helpful if the system is able to recognize the same patient with two different voucher numbers and recall the clinical history from previous voucher use. This can assist in determining appropriate patient management, but it may be difficult to make this information available to service providers without a sophisticated computer network.

Design of data collection forms is something of an art. The forms should be unambiguous and nonredundant, and they should include adequate space for responses (especially addresses). The check boxes and other spaces for responses should be aligned along the right-hand margin of the form, to facilitate data entry. Wherever possible, the form should occupy a single sheet of paper, even if this means using a larger sheet, a small font, or both, in order to prevent multiple sheets from becoming separated.

Perhaps the most common flaw in form design is making them too long. This wastes time and makes those filling out the forms less careful. Sometimes clinics gather more data than are required for the purposes of the scheme. These data need not be incorporated in the forms or reported in the information system. If possible, only data that will affect decision-making about the scheme should be solicited. The forms should be tested and retested before finalizing them and printing large quantities .

As a general rule, the voucher agency should receive a copy of all forms. Service providers will probably wish to keep a copy of the form for their records. Sometimes diagnostic service providers will require copies of at least parts of the clinic record. Multiple copies of forms can be produced cheaply using NCR (no carbon required) paper that prints through to the sheet below with the pressure of a pen.

Data Entry

Each form should be entered into a computerized database linking forms with voucher numbers. The data entry program can mimic the exact format of the form, with drop-down menus for multiple-choice responses, and it can perform consistency checks as the date is entered. The data entry phase can provide an additional opportunity to detect transfer of vouchers to indirect beneficiaries. Comparing names and surnames with those recorded at the time of distribution can be a first screen, but variations in spelling and the inclusion or exclusion of middle names can make it difficult to automate this process. If information such as the recipient's date of birth was recorded when the vouchers were distributed, it may be a better first screen for voucher transfer.

Using the Database to Run and Monitor the Program

What decisions and actions should the database assist? Many of these are related to monitoring and evaluation, discussed in chapter 7. In addition, the database should provide insights into the following:

- *Distribution strategies.* By providing voucher redemption rates for each voucher distributor, the information system identifies which are the most effective. This information can be used to create productivity incentives. The information system can also identify the distribution sites from which vouchers are most likely to be redeemed, and it can identify where they achieve the scheme's aims most cost-effectively.

- *Provider policies.* The database can identify which providers voucher bearers favor. This information can be used to drop ineffective providers by not renewing their contracts. If voucher bearers are expected to make more than one visit to a clinic, the proportion who fail to make a second visit may be used as an indicator of poor-quality care. Providers who provide such care can be dropped.

- *Provider remuneration.* The system can automatically generate monthly receipts for payments to providers.

- *Abuse.* The system can alert staff to possible counterfeiting, black market formation, collusion, or other types of fraud. The system can be programmed, for instance, to accept only voucher numbers that have been produced and distributed.

- *Reporting to funding agencies providing the subsidies.* The system can produce summaries of patient outcomes or service delivery outputs. If the voucher scheme is designed as an output-based assistance project, these outcomes or outputs will form the basis for invoicing the funding agency.

- *Storing medical records.* Where questions are raised about the management of individual patients, computerized databases can be used to quickly access records. An information system can also allow more than one staff member to access records at the same time.

- *Tracking cases and follow-up.* The information system is extremely useful as a way of flagging patients requiring follow-up or identifying individuals in response to queries from providers regarding their management.

CHECKLIST FOR VOUCHER DESIGN

It can be helpful to use a checklist when designing vouchers, to ensure that all of the issues surrounding the vouchers and their use have been considered and handled. Table 5-3 shows such a checklist.

Table 5-3. Checklist for Voucher Design

	Yes	No
Has the voucher agency been selected or created?		
Has a set of rules been drawn up to define who receives the vouchers, what the voucher entitles its bearer to, what the bearer must pay to the provider to use the voucher (if anything), who can participate in the scheme as service providers (and under what conditions), and what each provider will receive in payment from the voucher agency (and how payment is to be determined)?		
Have the voucher and promotional material been designed?		
Have the logistics systems (especially transport and communication) been fully worked out?		
Has a strategy for distributing the vouchers been selected?		
Have the mechanisms for paying contracted providers been determined?		
Has the information system been designed?		

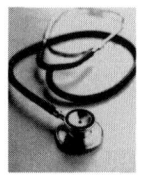

CHAPTER 6

IMPLEMENTING
A VOUCHER SCHEME

Successful implementation is not simply a matter of distributing vouchers and having them redeemed. It requires achieving the aims for which the subsidy scheme was created.

TENDERING FOR SERVICE PROVIDERS

If the number of service providers is limited—either because of the administrative costs involved or because of the desire to achieve potential economies of scale—some degree of competition can be retained by awarding the contract (or contracts) by public tender. Tendering for service providers allows the voucher agency to make a selection based on price and quality. In drawing up the announcement, it is essential to make the request for services as specific as possible to enable providers to price their services accurately and to avoid having to deal with a large number of unsuitable providers. To maximize the benefits of competition, it is important to encourage as many providers as possible to participate in the tendering. Advertising the tender, either in national newspapers or specialized periodicals, is one way to publicize the tender, but advertising can be expensive and some providers may miss the advertisement. Some providers may be reluctant to serve subsidized population groups for fear of lowering their status among their nonsubsidized clientele. Others may have preconceptions about slow and low payments (perhaps based on previous experience with the public sector). For these reasons, alternative strategies, such as mailings to clinics registered with the ministry of health or to individual providers, should also be considered.

In certain geographic settings or for certain highly specialized services, choosing providers may not be possible, and formal tendering is not appropriate. The existence of the subsidy scheme could encourage new providers to establish service provision in the area. If it does not, the voucher scheme can either use the only service provider available or contract services from providers outside the immediate area in which voucher recipients live in order to generate some competition.

Before contract negotiations begin, the provider policies established in the design stage need to be applied to the selection process. The process of selecting a provider must be totally transparent: all providers who expressed interest in participating must be told why they were or were not selected. Doing so will encourage them to participate in future tenders.

NEGOTIATING CONTRACTS

Negotiation is a process of communication in which two parties seek to arrive at a mutually satisfactory result on a matter of common concern. A mutually satisfactory result is necessary because each side depends on the other and both must live with the agreement. Box 6-1 provides some useful tips on negotiation.

Price

Price is one of the key points to be negotiated in a competitive voucher scheme. The voucher agency wants to keep the price as low as possible

Box 6-1.
Tips on Negotiation

- Listen carefully, be sensitive, and be quick to adapt to changing situations and to assess the impact of changing situations on the negotiation objectives.
- Avoid confrontation. Disagree with people politely. Use humor to defuse tension. Tolerate conflict while searching for agreement. Attack problems and sticking points, not individuals.
- Analyze and try to understand the interests and expectations of the other party.
- Prepare for the negotiating table by thinking through what your bottom line is (that is, the highest price you are prepared to pay and the terms of the contract that are not negotiable).
- Know the market well. Be aware of alternatives. If possible, prepare a draft contract for discussion.
- Sell your position.
- Where possible, deal with those who have the real decision-making power.
- Speak confidently and in a businesslike manner.
- Be honest and project honesty. Ploys and tricks may win the negotiation, but contract performance is likely to suffer.
- As a team, present a unified stance.
- Strive for long-term mutual satisfaction.
- Be prepared to make concessions and sacrifices that do not substantially affect the overall objectives but that demonstrate cooperation. Be creative, open minded, and flexible.
- Win results, not arguments.
- Apply objective standards to assess negotiation results.
- Emphasize win/win results of negotiation. Never suggest to the other party that it lost the negotiation.

without compromising service quality. One option is to accept the lowest price tendered. Another is to pay all providers a maximum benchmark price. A third is to attempt to negotiate lower prices from providers whose price tendered was close to the benchmark or from those who can offer the scheme something special (for example, a key location).

Quality Specifications

Technical and human quality specifications should be made clear; if accreditation is required (or offered), it should be discussed at this stage, before entering further into the negotiations. Lower- and middle-income countries may not have quality assurance schemes in place to guarantee a high and consistent level of quality of care. Guidance from the ministry of health may be available, but it may be inadequate and not up to date. In this case, policymakers should consider introducing their own accreditation scheme, by seeking technical assistance and building on the experience of other countries. The ministry of health may consider that accreditation is its prerogative, even if it is not currently offering it. Offering to extend the accreditation scheme to the public service could help assuage doubts and leave the entire health system with added value.

Minimum standards of care and patient management protocols should also be agreed on at this stage. Evidence-based management protocols— selected by experts in the voucher agency or by external consultants— should be the preferred choice. Some health service providers may not be up to date on these issues.

Ownership and Access Rights

It is important to establish and agree on ownership of laboratory specimens, X rays, and medical records; on who is to store them and for how long; and on who may have access to them in the future. It may be desirable for the voucher agency to retain intellectual property rights of all data for all studies and publications. Patient confidentiality must be respected at all times, but the voucher agency may want to request access to medical records for supervision or study purposes. If the voucher scheme incorporates a research component involving human subjects, it is essential to obtain approval from the appropriate bodies and, if necessary, informed consent from the patients.

CONTRACTING

Contracting is the process of formalizing an agreement that has been reached by negotiation. A written contract gives both parties the opportunity to express expectations and agree on outcomes. Sound contract design is a key element in a successful relationship with providers and therefore a prerequisite to the success of the program. Policymakers should not hesitate to include clauses in the contract that address issues of potential concern, provided that they do not compromise the scheme's flexibility. Box 6-2 provides an outline of the content of a typical contract.

Health care providers may not be accustomed to working under written contracts and may find the process threatening. It is therefore important to clarify that the main purpose of contracts is to set out and agree upon a set of rules that suit both parties. A contract should set out not only the provider's duties and commitments but also the purchaser's. For instance, the voucher agency may commit itself to train the provider's staff, to reimburse providers in a timely manner, to follow up specific cases, and so forth.

Contracts can be very simple, and they can evolve and change as the scheme goes on. It may make sense to establish a relatively short contract, especially for the first contract with a new provider, which can be renewed periodically if both sides are satisfied with each other's performance. Alternatively, the voucher agency may establish a trial period or make the contract conditional upon satisfaction with the provider's performance in the piloting phase. Once the methodology and logistics have been tried, the service provider may feel more relaxed about committing itself to a written contract, and the voucher agency has a better idea of the suitability of the provider.

TRAINING

All new programs involve a training component. In the case of voucher schemes, training can be needed for voucher agency staff, for contracted service providers, and for voucher distributors. What are the training needs at each level?

Box 6-2.
Elements in a Model Contract

1. The Agreement

1.1 *The parties.* Specifies who is the purchaser and who is the provider.

1.2 *The offer.* The provider says that he is prepared to provide the goods or services outlined in the contract (and its annexes) at a certain price. The annexes may include the provider's original offer, submitted as a bid during the tendering process. The offer is signed by the provider

1.3 *The acceptance.* The purchaser (the voucher agency) agrees to pay the provider according to the terms in the contract. The acceptance may also stipulate when the agreement comes into effect. The acceptance is signed by the voucher agency.

2. General Provisions

2.1 *Definitions.* Provided for words used as shorthand for longer titles (for example, the purchaser can be defined as whatever organization is purchasing the services) or for terms that may have an ambiguous interpretation (for example, *force majeure*).

2.2 *Law.* The parties agree to have the contract governed by the law in a particular jurisdiction.

2.3 *Communications.* Stipulates the mode (such as in writing) and language of communications to be used between the contracting parties.

3. The Purchaser

3.1 *Purchaser's representative.* Names the person authorized to represent the purchaser in dealings with the provider.

4. The Provider

4.1 *Provider's representative.* Names the person authorized to represent the provider in dealings with the purchaser.

4.2 *General obligations.* Can set down the provider's obligations with regard to the inputs it will need to complete the contract and their subsequent ownership.

Box 6-2. *Continued*

    4.3 *Subcontracting.* Can be used to restrict providers' rights to subcontract service provision to other entities.

5. Duration of Contract

    5.1 *Duration.* Specifies the date at which the contract ceases to be in force.

    5.2 *Extension.* Specifies the manner in which the duration of the contract can be extended.

6. Remedies

    6.1 *Remedying errors.* Used to assign responsibility (usually to the provider) to make good any faults due to poor equipment, consumables or standards of care, and so forth

    6.2 *Quality control.* Gives the purchaser the right to conduct checks on the quality of the services being delivered. The cost is usually assigned to the purchaser unless errors or faults attributable to the provider are uncovered.

7. Variations

Establishes procedures and rules for dealing with, for example, patients who do no fit the standard management protocol. Can allow for additional investigation and extra payments to the contractor. Can be used to give the voucher agency the flexibility to change the management protocol.

    7.1 *Right to vary.* Specifies who can make changes to the agreed upon services and under what conditions.

    7.2 *Value of variations.* Specifies what the provider will be paid for variations from the protocol.

    7.3 *Early warning.* Stipulates the warning that the parties must give each other for variation.

    7.4 *Right to claim.* Allows providers to claim for costs due to changes imposed by the voucher agency.

8. Contract prices and payments

    8.1 *Schedule of fees.* Gives the fees that the voucher agency agrees to pay the provider for specific services.

continued

Box 6-2. *Continued*

8.2 *Payment schedule.* States how often the voucher agency will make payments to the provider.

8.3 *Payment conditions.* Can stipulate conditions the provider must meet before being eligible to receive payment (for example, patient must sign receipt of laboratory results).

9. Default

9.1 *Default by the purchaser.* What happens in the event the purchaser fails to meet its obligations

9.2 *Default by the provider.* What happens in the event the provider fails to meet its obligations.

10. Risk and Responsibility

10.1 *Contractors' responsibilities.* Obligations, for example, to treat patients according to accepted ethical standards and to accept the consequences of medical negligence.

10.2 *Force majeure.* Unavoidable and unpredictable events not due to the other party. Medical misadventure may enter into this definition; the clause should establish what happens in these cases.

11. Resolution of Disputes

11.1 *Adjudication.* Names someone who can adjudicate a dispute that cannot be settled amicably and sets out how the adjudication will be performed.

11.2 *Notice of dissatisfaction.* Gives parties the opportunity to disagree with results of adjudication before it becomes binding and to take the process to arbitration.

11.3 *Arbitration.* Can provide an alternative mechanism for settling disputes without recourse to legal action.

12. Appendices

Provides detail on the goods or services to be provided (for example, the detailed patient management protocols). The contract should state that these form an integral part of the agreement. The appendices can also set out detailed rules for arbitration, adjudication, and other aspects of the contract.

Training within the Voucher Agency

For the voucher agency, the training required will depend on the existing skills mix of the staff. Training should be tailored to the specific tasks the agency is required to perform. These will normally include tendering, negotiating contracts with service providers, monitoring contract performance, designing and running information systems, evaluating the program, accounting and paying contractors, training providers and voucher distributors, designing promotional and client information materials (including the voucher itself), and dealing with complaints and queries from voucher recipients. Some of these tasks (such as the design of promotional materials) can and probably should be contracted out to organizations that specialize in them. It will often, however, be necessary to have at least one staff member with a good knowledge of the health problem being addressed and the interventions used. Some schemes place restrictions on service providers, requiring that only staff who have taken part in training workshops can care for voucher patients, for example, or that only female staff can conduct gynecological examinations. If other voucher schemes are in operation in the country, it would be beneficial for them to provide some training, as there is no substitute for hands-on experience.

Training Service Providers

Training for service providers could include instruction on how to fill out the forms correctly and how to return vouchers for payment, as well as explanations of management protocols, contractual obligations, and payment procedures. If there are aspects of the management protocol that are novel or technically challenging, it may be necessary to provide training in these areas, too.

The training of receptionists should not be overlooked. The receptionist is usually the first service provider the voucher bearer meets. The validity of the voucher needs to be acknowledged immediately to avoid any embarrassment for the patient. The agency may have negotiated preferential treatment for voucher-bearing patients, which is something the reception staff often control. The training of receptionists is in the interests of the provider, as a bad experience of one patient may deter attendance by others. Emphasizing the importance of treating voucher bearers with respect and courtesy and maintaining their privacy can play a key role in preventing voucher bearers from feeling stigmatized.

Training Voucher Distributors

Voucher distributors are usually the first point of contact between the scheme and the target population. They therefore play a key role in explaining what benefits the voucher offers (and does not offer), in convincing the recipient of its legitimacy, and in answering any questions or doubts patients may have about the scheme. Some of the most difficult-to-reach groups (indigenous populations, drug users, commercial sex workers) tend to be suspicious of outsiders and require sensitive handling. Social anthropologists, who are trained in these skills, are well-placed to train voucher distributors. It is important to remember that training is an ongoing activity. Staffs change, new service providers and voucher distributors enter the scheme, and policies change. Periodic training is therefore worthwhile.

PILOTING

Piloting is a crucial step in implementing any program. It is especially important for voucher schemes, where several different parties and a wide range of activities are often involved. Piloting provides a chance to try out all strategies and their logistics and to modify them based on the results. It is important to resist the temptation of excluding small logistical or organizational steps from piloting.

All components of a program need not be tested at the same time. Piloting of the voucher design, for instance, can be done at the beginning of the program, before any other stage is commenced. The scheme's educational material should also be tested early on, as well as its information systems. Time limits should be set on piloting, so that it does not continue indefinitely in an attempt to perfect the system. Restricting the piloting to a geographic area and to a specific number of vouchers can also help make the process more efficient.

Piloting can result in the exclusion of certain providers and the inclusion of more appropriate ones. It can also result in dramatic changes in strategies. Such change need not be viewed as a failure but as a chance to rethink different processes to ensure the program's success. The example in box 6-3 describes how piloting led to a significant change in the design of a voucher when a scheme from one country was tested in another.

Piloting is not complete until the results have been formally assessed and acted on. A time needs to be set aside to consider which aspects of the scheme's design worked and which did not. This is the time to translate poorly performing strategies into changes to the scheme. It is vital to resist committing the program to a fixed set of strategies, even if the funding agency applies pressure to do so. Once again, flexibility is the key to success.

Box 6-3.
How Piloting Can Lead to Changes in Strategy

The El Salvador cervical cancer program was to implement many of the same strategies successfully tried out in the Nicaraguan program, including the advertising material. However, when the project's logo was tested in El Salvador, program designers discovered that what was considered feminine and discrete in Nicaragua was interpreted as offensive in El Salvador. The nude woman in the Nicaraguan logo became a dressed woman in the Salvadoran logo.

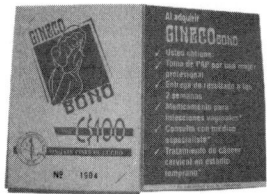
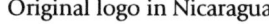
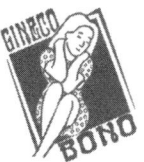

Original logo in Nicaragua   Logo adapted for El Salvador

The voucher distribution in El Salvador was going to make use of traditional birth attendants, in the hope that their relationship with older women would facilitate the distribution. However, when this component of the program was pilot tested, traditional birth attendants managed to distribute only a handful of vouchers. The strategy of voucher distribution had to be rethought. Currently, vouchers are being distributed by community health workers.

INSTITUTIONALIZING

Because of their novelty, voucher schemes are often introduced with significant levels of external technical assistance. Institutionalizing is about making the transition from an experimental initiative, or "project," to a sustained, ongoing health program. Part of this institutionalization process is about weaning off of technical assistance. Another part is about establishing norms for the various activities (such as contracting new clinics or paying for redeemed vouchers) that are repeated. A third element is a conscious search for ways to minimize ongoing costs.

Experience has shown that the institutionalization phase must be taken as a conscious step. It is otherwise all too easy to allow the ad hoc approach that typifies (and indeed helps) new initiatives to continue indefinitely. Although it is not always possible, ensuring that trained staff stay on the job is a key element to ensure a smooth transition, even if it means increasing their salaries.

A danger in institutionalizing a program can be the fact that, in an effort to simplify and streamline all aspects of the scheme, the flexibility of the program is compromised. Remaining project staff must be left some room to maneuver, conceptually and operationally, in order to respond adequately to new threats and opportunities faced by the voucher scheme. Retaining access to ongoing but occasional technical assistance in these instances could be budgeted for.

SCALING UP

Scaling up is a process that can occur at least twice in the implementation of a voucher scheme. The first occasion occurs when the pilot testing ends and the project is applied to the full target population. This full implementation phase does not necessarily imply nationwide coverage. Voucher schemes often begin as small innovative projects aimed at serving the needs of relatively small and geographically limited population groups. If the scheme is perceived as having been successful, there is therefore often a subsequent stage or stages of scaling up to cover a much wider proportion of the population—by expanding either geographically or in scope to cover new target groups.

Scaling up can greatly improve the efficiency of a voucher scheme, since there are certain relatively fixed administrative costs inherent in the use of vouchers, such as the need for a voucher agency. But when voucher schemes begin as small projects, they often start up in the most favorable settings, where there are a wide range of potential service providers willing to compete for contracts. As they expand, the settings may become less conducive to competitive schemes, the costs of transport and communications tend to rise, and the quality of services may decline. These factors can easily undermine the efficiency gains of greater scale.

As the scale increases, the number of institutions that become involved tends to increase. Until voucher schemes form part of the orthodoxy of health development assistance, merely securing agreement to introduce a voucher scheme can meet resistance.

The distribution of tasks within the voucher agency tends to become more specialized as a scheme is scaled up. Although this may mean that specific tasks are performed more efficiently, there remains a need for someone—perhaps the scheme's coordinator—to retain a broad vision of how the scheme is operating.

As the program expands, some of the systems initially established by the voucher agency—computer databases, communications, contract negotiation skills, transport—may begin to fail as they reach the limits of their capacities. These problems can be overcome by upgrading and expanding technologies and training, but the process of doing so can be time consuming.

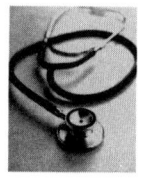

CHAPTER 7

MONITORING AND EVALUATING A VOUCHER PROGRAM

Monitoring is the process of routinely gathering information to determine whether something is meeting expectations. Evaluation, in its broadest sense, is the process of assessing something or making a judgment. House (1980) sees evaluation as a process that leads to a judgment about the worth of something, a settled opinion that usually leads to a decision to act in a certain way. Clearly, there is overlap between monitoring and evaluation, but a distinction can be made. Monitoring is an ongoing activity, whereas evaluation is carried out periodically. Evaluation necessarily involves judgments, whereas monitoring can be merely observation. Monitoring is normally carried out by people responsible for running the system. Evaluation is often conducted by people who do not have direct responsibility for running the system.

Monitoring and evaluation of the voucher scheme begin before the first voucher is distributed. It starts at the design stage, by careful consideration of what activities and outputs need to be monitored, what information will be needed to monitor them, and how that information can be gathered in the most economical and timely fashion without compromising quality.

One of the beauties of voucher schemes is the ease with which monitoring and evaluation can be performed. This is because the vouchers themselves define discrete units for which individual processes and outcomes can be traced and measured.

Monitoring and evaluation involve the following tasks:

- Determine what aspects of the voucher scheme need to be monitored.

- Determine how and when these aspects should be monitored.

- Establish the necessary systems for conducting the monitoring.

- Conduct the monitoring.

- Determine the basis upon which the voucher scheme should be evaluated.

- Determine how and when evaluation should be carried out.

- Conduct the evaluation.

Figure 7-1 lists the eight areas that should be addressed in developing monitoring systems and evaluating the scheme. They are not presented in any particular order.

MONITORING SERVICE QUALITY

Quality includes technical quality, which affects the scheme's ability to improve health, and human quality, which relates to patients' satisfaction with the services rendered. In both cases, monitoring involves three steps: setting and reviewing verifiable standards, measuring quality, and reviewing results.

In setting standards, policymakers have at least three options. One is to allow providers to set the standards themselves. A second is to impose externally set standards on providers. The third is for the voucher agency and providers to negotiate and agree on a set of standards. The advantage of

Figure 7-1. Monitoring and Evaluating the Voucher Program

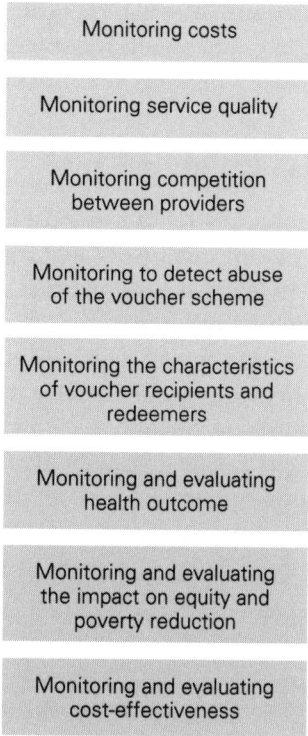

the first strategy is that it gives providers a stake in the process, which can make them more receptive to improving quality. The advantage of the second option is that standards can be chosen that are known to be adequate for achieving the expected health gains or patient satisfaction. The third strategy, which is one that voucher schemes and other contract-based programs lend themselves to, should have the advantages of both of the first two options.

Monitoring Technical Standards

To be objective, the measurement of quality must be neutral and well publicized. If the voucher scheme incorporates accreditation, the process needs to be repeated periodically. Certain health services need more supervision than others, particularly those for which performance is known to vary widely (such as sputum microscopy for tuberculosis and cervical cytology). One policy is to require accreditation of all new providers. For laboratory-based care, samples can be regularly doubled-checked at a different institution and comparisons of performance made over time.

Monitoring the Human Quality of Care

Measurement of the human quality of care poses less of a problem. Patients can bear testimony to the quality of care they receive. They can provide objective information (such as waiting times) and subjective indicators of satisfaction. Patients can be interviewed as they leave a facility (sometimes it may even be sufficient to interview non-voucher-bearing patients), but the presence of an interviewer outside the clinic may annoy the provider or change his or her treatment of patients. Tracing patients at the point at which their vouchers were originally distributed may be a better strategy and one that allows people who had not used their vouchers to be interviewed. Respondents who have used the voucher are normally willing to share their experience and take the time to participate in the evaluation.

"Mystery Patients"

Another alternative for monitoring human quality (and even some aspects of technical quality) is the use of "mystery patients." These are people employed by the voucher agency who pose as voucher-bearing patients. Providers can be warned in advance that they can expect such visits as part of quality monitoring (and the use of mystery patients can be written into the contract). Mystery patients can report back on all aspects of care: whether the premises were clean and tidy, the receptionist was polite, waiting times were acceptable, doctors and nurses discriminated against the patient, the procedures performed were fully explained, and so forth. Mystery patients can be very useful if given thorough guidance in advance, but their ability to assess the technical quality of care is usually quite limited, unless they are health professionals themselves.

Field Visits and Facility Inspections

Voucher agency staff should make periodic unannounced visits to the health facility and speak with staff to gather their views. These visits can be used to ensure that all equipment is still available and working properly and that forms are being filled out correctly. The staff member can accompany a voucher bearer to observe the full process of care.

Interpreting Findings

Random fluctuations and normal error in measurement can account for some variation in results. One should therefore take action only when these results lie outside the limits of what might be expected as a result of such variation. The frequency with which one reviews the quality indicators is a matter of judgment. If monitoring is done too infrequently, one may miss some serious problems with service quality that could affect the impact of the scheme. Monitoring too frequently increases the administrative burden, however, as well as the random variation.

MONITORING COMPETITION AMONG PROVIDERS

One of the more useful process indicators that can be monitored is the degree of competition in the scheme. If there is little competition among providers, many of the benefits of the voucher scheme, such as improved quality and cost containment, may not materialize. The degree of competition within the voucher scheme will change over time, as providers enter and leave and as providers' shares of the total number of vouchers change.

A widely accepted measure of the degree of competition is the Herfindahl-Hirschmann index (HHI) of concentration (box 7-1). HHI levels above 1,000 indicate moderate market concentration; HHI levels above 1,800 are considered highly concentrated (U.S. Department of Justice and Federal Trade Commission 1997).

One must use these indices with some caution, for several reasons. First, there may be competition simply to enter the scheme, but providers who are not selected do not enter into the calculations. Second, even with a large number of providers, each with a small market share, competition may not be perfect. Geographic location, to name just one factor, will also affect competition, because voucher bearers may prefer to go to a clinic of worse quality if it means less traveling. Third, in fully subsidized schemes, providers are not competing on price for their share, since the price has already been negotiated with the voucher agency. Notwithstanding these limitations, the HHI does illustrate the importance to competition of hav-

Box 7-1.
Calculating the Herfindahl-Hirschmann Index of
Concentration

The Herfindahl-Hirschmann index is calculated using the following four steps:

1. Write down the names of all providers in the first column.
2. In the next column, write down the proportion of the total number of vouchers redeemed with each provider during the period
   monitored.
3. In the third column, write down the square of each of those per-
   centages.
4. Add up all of the numbers in the third column. This is the HHI.

Sample Calculation of the HHI of Concentration

Clinic	Share of vouchers (percent)	Score
A	30	900
B	25	625
C	20	400
D	15	225
E	10	100
HHI	2,450	

ing as many providers as possible and a relatively even distribution of
market share. This should be borne in mind when making decisions about
adding or dropping providers from the scheme.

MONITORING TO DETECT ABUSE OF THE VOUCHER
SCHEME

Voucher schemes can be abused or misused in a variety of ways, including
counterfeiting, collusion between providers and voucher bearers or distributors, black market sales, bribery and kickbacks, overservicing,

provider moral hazard, adverse selection, and cream-skimming (cherry-picking).

Counterfeiting

The risk of counterfeiting and development of a black market for vouchers is highest if the vouchers have a high monetary value or if they subsidize a highly sought service. This risk should have been considered during the design phase and measures taken to keep it to a minimum. However, in some cases it may be better (and cheaper) simply to monitor the scheme carefully to detect abuse or misuse as soon as it occurs.

If a computerized information system has been developed, it can automatically flag redeemed vouchers that have not yet been printed or distributed (or ones for which the check digits do not tally). In addition, the system can match the voucher number with the geographic area in which it was distributed or with the name of the patient to whom it was given (if this information was collected and recorded). It may also be desirable to monitor for counterfeiting by providers. It is sensible to share at least the obvious anti-counterfeiting measures with providers and ask them to check vouchers for these. The less obvious checks for counterfeiting should be kept secret by the voucher agency for its own use. This is perhaps most important where the voucher has little or no monetary value, since the only people who could then readily convert them into cash would be service providers.

Collusion

A slightly different situation arises when there is collusion between the voucher distributor and health service providers: voucher distributors may give in to the temptation to come to an agreement with one or more service providers to give them vouchers in exchange for part of the earnings. The service provider could then ensure that all (or the majority) of the vouchers are "redeemed" at his or her clinic and could return them without providing services. This fraud may be detected if there is a sudden change in the proportion of vouchers returned from a particular provider. Visiting and interviewing a proportion of patients can also uncover such scams. It is unlikely, however, that many health service providers would stoop to such actions. Apart from the ill repute they would earn if caught—as well as the possible criminal charges—they would still have to ensure that the names of recipients submitted by the voucher distributors match those on the forms they send to the voucher agency. Inventing patients requires even more work, not to mention the difficulty of obtaining laboratory specimens if these are required.

Black Markets

If the benefits provided by the voucher are of high value and the vouchers are widely demanded, a black market for them may develop. It may be worth monitoring to detect the existence and size of such a market. Until it appears, or unless it becomes significant in scope, it may not be necessary to do more than monitor the situation. If black market trading becomes a serious problem, some of the other measures to enforce non-transferability may be necessary (see box 5-2). Printing "no monetary value" on the voucher, as well as mentioning that in any educational or social marketing campaign, may also help.

Dishonesty within the Voucher Agency

The voucher agency or its staff may receive bribes in return for contracting with certain providers or agreeing to higher than necessary voucher payments. The risk of this form of abuse can be reduced by having strict rules regarding contracting with providers and by setting a single price for all providers. Such rules can undermine the flexibility of the voucher scheme, but they may be necessary to yield adequate transparency. An important monitoring measure that should be taken is external financial audit.

Overservicing

Where the voucher agency pays providers different sums based on patient characteristics, providers may be tempted to shift patients from lower- to higher-paying categories, even if it means providing services the patients do not merit according to the management protocol. This possibility, called "moral hazard" (or "overservicing"), is well-known to health insurance schemes. Monitoring costs is one way of detecting or at least screening for it. Another way to monitor for provider moral hazard is to periodically review a sample of cases from each provider that qualified for the higher payments, to ensure that it meets the established criteria.

Adverse Selection

Adverse selection is most likely to occur where vouchers incorporate some element of risk spreading. For example, if a voucher covering the cost of both screening and treatment for a disease is sold, those who are free of the disease usually subsidize those who are not. This means that there is an incentive for patients diagnosed elsewhere to purchase a voucher and receive the treatment at a subsidized cost. This raises the average cost per voucher and can make the screening and treatment vouchers uncompetitive with screening alone. Thus individuals will tend to pay to be tested elsewhere and will buy the voucher only if they are found to be positive. The result can be a collapse of the scheme. To avoid this eventuality, individuals who know that they have a disease could be prohibited from purchasing the voucher, but in many cases it is impossible to enforce. What could help in this case is making it clear to the voucher distributor (or seller) that vouchers should not be given away to people who are known to have the disease.

If the main aim of the voucher scheme is to detect and treat a disease, to subsidize the poor, or both, adverse selection need not be a major concern. Indeed, it may represent an improvement in technical efficiency if those most at risk of a disease are most likely to use their voucher. Where diagnosis outside the voucher scheme is not reliable, adverse selection becomes less of a risk, because many of those seeking prepaid treatment may not actually have the disease and will therefore not require treatment (see box 7-2).

Cream-Skimming (Cherry-Picking)

Cream-skimming, sometimes known as cherry-picking, is a form of provider adverse selection in which voucher bearers whose costs are likely to exceed the payment received from the voucher agency are excluded or obstructed from redeeming their vouchers while patients whose costs are likely to be lower are actively encouraged to redeem their vouchers. Instead of competing to attract voucher-bearing patients, providers compete to attract low-cost patients and off-load high-cost patients onto other providers.

Cream-skimming is relatively easy to detect by examining the profile of patients at each of the clinics in relation to the services (and hence costs) they receive from the providers. It can be addressed by weighting pay-

---

Box 7-2.
Improving Targeting through Adverse Selection

A scheme in Nicaragua sold vouchers with prepaid screening for
and treatment of cervical cancer. The scheme allowed women who
had previously been diagnosed by Pap smear as having a high-
grade lesion to purchase the voucher, because the quality of smear
diagnosis outside the scheme was generally so poor that many of
these patients did not actually have these lesions. However, since
there was considerable variation in the quality of cytological
screening outside the scheme, some patients did benefit from adverse selection. If the quality of screening nationwide rose to the
standards within the program (which is possible, since it initiated
an external quality assurance scheme for all cytologists), then adverse selection may become more of a concern. In contrast, for fully or highly subsidized schemes, adverse selection helps improve
targeting and therefore the program's efficiency at achieving its
aims.

---

ments according to the patient profile (individually or across the facility as
a whole), but care must be taken to ensure that this differential payment
strategy does not create provider moral hazard.

MONITORING THE CHARACTERISTICS OF VOUCHER
RECIPIENTS AND REDEEMERS

Knowing who received the vouchers is useful for measuring the efficiency
of the distribution system at targeting priority groups. This information
can also be used to identify the best distributors. Monitoring can reveal
who distributed the most vouchers and who best targeted the priority
groups. Together with information on who has redeemed vouchers, this
information can reveal who has the highest redemption rates. Distributors
who distribute the most vouchers may not be the ones who have the most
vouchers redeemed at service providers. The difference may depend on
how good they are at explaining what the vouchers are for and why they

should be used. This information can be used as the basis for providing incentives to distributors. For instance, a prize or special recognition could be offered to the distributor with the highest redemption rate among priority groups.

Monitoring these characteristics can also serve another important purpose. It is often valuable to understand why some people choose not to use their vouchers. This knowledge can help the voucher agency design strategies to improve redemption rates. Small changes in the way the scheme is designed or promoted may greatly improve redemption rates. In particular, the voucher agency will want to know whether recipients are fully aware of the benefits the voucher offers. Of course, it may be that nonredeemers are a self-selected subgroup of low-priority individuals. Qualitative as well as quantitative data must be collected to understand why recipients are not redeeming their vouchers. Keeping a record of the names and addresses of voucher recipients makes it possible to go back to interview samples of those who chose not to redeem their vouchers and thus identify any unforeseen barriers to service uptake.

MONITORING AND EVALUATING HEALTH OUTCOMES

Outcomes include reducing inequalities in health, compensating for the presence of externalities, and addressing the distortions caused by incomplete and asymmetrical information. In the case of externalities, the problem is often one of underconsumption of services that (for example) lead to lower population growth rates or reduce the transmission of communicable disease. The impact of subsidies should therefore be measured in terms of how well they achieve specific outcomes, such as lower birth rates and transmission of infectious disease.

Program evaluation is often complicated by the difficulty of determining whether changes in outcome indicators are attributable to the program or to other extraneous factors. In this regard, voucher schemes have some advantages over other ways of delivering subsidies, because one can pinpoint who has been a beneficiary of the program and who has not. It therefore becomes relatively simple to establish what goods or services each beneficiary (or at least a sample of them) received. Evaluating the scheme's impact becomes a matter of determining what the outcome would have been for these individuals had they not received vouchers. Three different approaches can be used. One is to estimates how these individuals would have fared had the voucher scheme not been introduced. Another is to compare outcomes among voucher recipients and nonrecipients. The third is to ask voucher recipients what they would have done had the voucher scheme not existed and to speculate on what the outcome would have been. None of these approaches is perfect, but all give a better indication of impact than merely measuring outcomes among voucher recipients alone.

Subsidies are justified for the treatment and prevention of communicable disease because avoiding or reducing the duration of an infection in one person reduces the risk of others contracting the disease. This makes it difficult to determine the true impact of subsidies. It is difficult to know how many infections are avoided for every one treated or how many are prevented by immunization among those not immunized because of herd immunity. Sophisticated mathematical models are being developed to help answer these questions, but they are not yet used regularly in program evaluation. In practice, one is often limited to quantifying the impact on voucher recipients and making assumptions about the downstream benefits of these outcomes.

MONITORING AND EVALUATING THE IMPACT ON EQUITY AND POVERTY REDUCTION

Ideally, one would like to know the number or proportion of voucher recipients whom the scheme protects from becoming impoverished or the reduction in income inequalities in health outcomes. This is known as poverty impact analysis. In practice, these outcomes can be very difficult to measure because of the need to simultaneously measure changes in the health status of subgroups within a population as well as within the population as a whole and to demonstrate that differences among subgroups were caused by the program.

Benefit incidence analysis seeks to quantify how program subsidies are distributed across socioeconomic classes.[1] It seeks to find out how well the voucher scheme has targeted resources to the poor and whether it has done so more effectively than existing subsidy schemes. The first of these aims can be achieved by documenting the socioeconomic profile of

---

[1] The term "incidence" is used here in a quite different sense from that used in epidemiology, where it is a measure of the frequency of occurrence of a disease event.

voucher scheme beneficiaries and comparing it with the socioeconomic profile of the general population. The second requires data on the existing benefit incidence of government spending on health. These data may be obtained by documenting the socioeconomic profile of a sample of health service users weighted by spending on services to each (for example, hospital users consume a much higher level of government subsidies than ambulatory care users and may have quite a different socioeconomic profile).

An even simpler way of evaluating a program is to examine the service outputs (for example, receipt and utilization of vouchers) in terms of the socioeconomic profile of the beneficiaries. Doing so avoids the need to quantify the value of these outputs in terms of the level of subsidy going into each. If the same socioeconomic indicators have been measured in other subsidy schemes or for government health expenditure generally, a judgment can be made about the equity impact of the scheme.

Irrespective of the type of analysis, monitoring and evaluation of equity must compare differences in outcomes by socioeconomic status. Without a consistent summary measure, confusion can arise, because differences or changes over time can be caused by either variation in the socioeconomic status of the populations being compared or by variation in the distribution of health outcomes among them. This issue can be addressed by using appropriate summary measures, such as concentration coefficients or the index of relative inequality (Wagstaff, Paci, and Van Doorslaer 1991).

Some measurement of income or socioeconomic status among program participants is required. If one wishes to make comparisons with the population as a whole, the measures or indicators of socioeconomic status should be ones that have been applied in censuses or surveys nationwide. Income is perhaps the best indicator of socioeconomic status, but measuring it in developing countries is fraught with difficulties and rarely practical. Measuring household expenditure is often more reliable, but it is also too time consuming for routine data collection. A better alternative is to record the same proxy indicators of socioeconomic status used in censuses and representative population surveys. These may include educational level, house construction materials, number of household members per bedroom, and certain key household assets.

These data can be collected either at the time the vouchers are distributed or at the point of service provision. The advantage of collecting the data when the vouchers are distributed is that it permits the socioeconomic status of voucher redeemers and nonredeemers to be compared. Moreover, if distribution is done house to house, the distributor can observe or verify house construction materials and asset ownership, if these are used as indicators. People may be suspicious or embarrassed to disclose details regarding their housing or income status to a young person who may be one of their neighbors, however.

MONITORING AND EVALUATING COST-EFFECTIVENESS

Evaluation of cost-effectiveness of the program is one of the most difficult enterprises in public health. Vouchers simplify this process, however, often making it possible to accurately measure both costs and project-specific outcomes. If costs and outcomes are monitored, monitoring cost-effectiveness becomes simply a matter of calculating the ratio of positive outcomes to the cost of the program. Problems arise, however, when one wishes to compare alternative subsidy schemes or the status quo, because accurate information on costs and outcomes is much harder to come by.

REFERENCES

Angrist, J., E. Bettinger, E. Bloom, E. King, and M. Kremer. 2001. *Vouchers for Private Schooling in Colombia: Evidence from a Randomized Natural Experiment*. Boston: National Bureau of Economic Research.

—. 1995. "Sexual Health and STDs: An Avenue to HIV Prevention Services." *AIDS Information Exchange (U.S. Conference of Mayors)* 12: 6–8.

Astin, A.W. 1992. "Educational 'Choice': Its Appeal May Be Illusory." *Sociology of Education* 65(4): 255–260.

Bennell, P. 1997. *Vocational Education and Training in Zimbabwe: The Role of Private Sector Provision in the Context of Economic Reform*. Institute of Development Studies Research Report, University of Sussex, United Kingdom.

Bertsch, E.F. 1992. "A Voucher System that Enables Persons with Severe Mental Illness to Purchase Community Support Services." *Hospital Community Psychiatry* 4311: 1109–1113.

Birkhead, G.S, C.W. Lebaron, P. Parsons, J.C. Grabau, L. Barr-Gale, J. Fuhrman, S. Brooks, J. Rosenthal, S.C. Hadler, and D.L. Morse. 1995. "The Immunization of Children Enrolled in the Special Supplemental Food Program for Women, Infants, and Children (WIC): The Impact of Different Strategies." *Journal of the American Medical Association* 2744: 312–316.

Blanck, P., L. Clay, J. Schmeling, M. Morris, and H. Ritchie. 2002. "Applicability of the ADA to 'Ticket to Work' Employment Networks." *Behav Sci Law* 206: 621–636.

BONOSOL. 2003. Available at www.Bonosol.Bo.

Bono ISAPRE 2003. Available at www.andueza.Cl.

Bono AUGE 2003. Available at www.Fonasa.Gov.Cl.

Borghi, J., A. Gorter, P. Sandiford, and Z. Segura. 2003. "The Cost-Effectiveness of a Voucher Scheme to Reduce Sexually Transmitted Infections in Sex Workers and Their Clients: The Case of Managua, Nicaragua." Paper presented at the Fourth World Congress of the International Health Economics Association, San Francisco.

Bosselaar, H., and R. Prins 2001. *Return to Work of Disabled Persons: The Dutch Reintegration Voucher.* Meccano, Netherlands: European Employment Observatory.

Calero, C. 2003a. *El Salvador: Cervical Cancer Prevention for Poor Rural Women.* Instituto Centro Americano de la Salud. Managua, Nicaragua.

—. 2003b. *Questionnaire for the World Bank Study on Voucher Schemes for Health.* Instituto Centro Americano de la Salud. Managua, Nicaragua.

Caram, M. 2002. "Voucher Program on Reproductive Health: Profamilia Project Report." Profamilia. Santo Domingo, Dominican Republic.

Cernada, G., and L.P. Chow. 1969. "The Coupon System." *American Journal of Public Health* 59 (12): 147-166.

—. 1970. "The Coupon System." In *The Taiwan Family Planning Reader,* ed. George P. Cernada, 147–166. Taichung: Chinese Center for International Training in Family Planning.

Cohen, D.K., and E. Farrar. 1977. "Power to the Parents? The Story of Education Vouchers." *Public Interest* 48 (1): 72–97.

Culyer, A.J., J.W. Posnett, A.J. Culyer, A. Maynard, and J. Posnett, eds. 1990. *Competition in Health Care: Reforming The NHS. Vol. 1, Hospital Behavior and Competition.* London: Macmillan.

Dole, G.F., and P.A. Carney. 1998. "Characteristics of Underserved Women Who Did and Those Who Did Not Use A Free/Low-Cost Voucher as Part of a Mammography Screening Program." *Journal of Cancer Education* 13 (2): 102–107.

Du, K., K. Zhang, and S. Tang S. 1999. "Summary of 'A Draft Report on a MCHPAF Study in China.'" Poverty Net Library. Available at poverty.worldbank.org/library/.

Friedman, M. 1962. *Capitalism and Freedom.* Chicago: University of Chicago Press.

Friedman, J., and D.H. Weinberg. 1982. *The Economics of Housing Vouchers.* New York: Academic Press.

Galasso, E., M. Ravallion, and A. Salvia. 2001. "Assisting the Transition form Workfare to Work Argentina's Proempleo Experiment." Poverty Net Library. Available at poverty.worldbank.org/library/.

Gauri, V. 1998. *School Choice in Chile: Two Decades of Educational Reform.* Pittsburgh, PA: University of Pittsburgh Press.

Gauri, V., and A. Vawda. 2003. "Vouchers for Basic Education in Developing Countries, A Principal-Agent Perspective." Policy Research Working Paper 3005, World Bank, Washington, DC.

Gorter, A. 2002. *A Voucher Scheme for Adolescents in Nicaragua to Improve the Uptake of Reproductive Health Services*. Project report for DfID (Department for International Development), Instituto CentroAmericano de la Salud, Managua, Nicaragua.

—. 2003. "Review Paper on Evidence for Using Competitive Voucher Schemes and Related Methods for Ensuring Young People Have Access to Health Service Interventions Designed to Prevent or Provide Care for HIV/AIDS." Background paper prepared for the Consultation on the Health Services Response to the Prevention and Care of HIV/AIDS among Young People, organized by WHO with UNICEF, UNFPA, UNAIDS, and Youthnet, Montreux, Switzerland.

Gorter, A., Z. Segura, and P. Sandiford. 2002. "Competitive Voucher Schemes for Better Health for Vulnerable Populations and Poor." Invited clinic and presentation at the Discussion Forum on Private Provision of Health Services in Developing Countries, World Bank, Washington DC.

Green, J., W. Howell, and P. Peterson. 1997. "An Evaluation of the Cleveland Scholarship Program." Occasional Paper, Harvard University, Program in Education Policy and Governance, Cambridge, MA. Available at http://www.schoolchoices.org/roo/cleveland1.htm.

Green, J.P., P.E. Peterson, and J. Du. 1997. "Effectiveness of School Choice: The Milwaukee Experiment." Occasional Paper 97, Harvard University, Program in Education Policy and Governance, Cambridge, MA.

Gwatkin, D.R. 2000. "The Current State of Knowledge about Targeting Health Programs to Reach the Poor." World Bank, Washington, DC.

Hammett, T.M., D.C. Des Jarlais, W. Liu, D. Ngu, and N. Son. 2002. "A Cross-Border HIV Prevention Intervention for Injection Drug Users (IDUs) in Ning Ming Country Guangxi Province, China and Lang Son Province, Vietnam." Paper presented at the 14th International AIDS Conference, Barcelona, Spain.

Higgins, S.T., A.J. Budney, W.K. Bickel, F.E. Foerg, R. Donham, and G.J. Badger. 1994. "Incentives Improve Outcome: Outpatient Behavioral Treatment of Cocaine Dependence." *Arch Gen Psychiatry* 51: 568–576.

Higgins, S.T., S.M. Alessi, and R.L. Dantona 2002. "Voucher-Based Incentives: A Substance Abuse Treatment Innovation." *Addict Behav* 276: 887–910.

House, E.R 1980. *Evaluating with Validity*. Beverly Hills, CA: Sage.

House of Commons. 1996. *Proceedings of the British Parliament*. November 13. London.

Hsieh, C.-T., and M. Urquiola. 2002. "When Schools Compete, How Do They Compete? An Assessment of Chile's Nationwide School Voucher Program."

Occasional Paper No. 43, National Center for the Study of Privatization in Education, New York.

Kent County Council Education Department. 1978. *Education Vouchers in Kent: A Feasibility Study for The Education Department of The Kent County Council.* Kent County Council, Maidstone, United Kingdom.

Kiefe, C.I., S.V. Mckay, A. Halevy, and B.A. Brody. 1994. "Is Cost a Barrier to Screening Mammography for Low-Income Women Receiving Medicare Benefits? A Randomized Trial." *Arch Intern Med* 15411: 1217–1224.

King, E., P. Ozarem, and D. Wohlgemuth. 1998. "Central Mandates and Local Incentives: The Colombia Education Voucher Program." Paper No. 6, Working Paper Series on Impact Evaluation of Education Reforms, World Bank, Development Research Group, Washington, DC.

Knowles, James C. 2000. *Consultant's Report of Technical Assistance Provided to the BDD Sustainability Component of the Safe Motherhood Project.* Draft consultant's report to the World Bank for the Indonesian Safe Motherhood Project.

Koumans, E.H., K. Barker, M. Massanga, R.V. Hawkins, P. Somse, K.A. Parker, and J. Moran. 2003. "Patient-Led Partner Referral Enhances Sexually Transmitted Disease Service Delivery in Two Towns in the Central African Republic." Int *J STD AIDS* 106: 376–382.

Luft, H.S. 1984. "On the Use of Vouchers for Medicare." *Milbank Memorial Fund Quarterly / Health and Society,* 62, No.2: 237–250.

Marchant, T., J.A. Schellenberg, T. Edgar, R. Nathan, S. Abdulla, O. Mukasa, H. Mponda, and C. Lengeler. 2002. "Socially Marketed Insecticide-Treated Nets Improve Malaria and Anemia in Pregnancy in Southern Tanzania." *Trop Med Int Health* 72: 149–58.

Migrant Health Programs Dick Bohrer Paper. 2001. *Observations and Recommendations on Migrant Health Programs to the Office of Migrant Health: Version 5 Draft Incorporating the Observations, Critiques, and Contributions of the MHP Action Team.* Office of Migrant Health, Bureau of Primary Health Care, Bethesda, Maryland.

Mookherji, S. 2003. *Questionnaire for the World Bank Study on Voucher Schemes for Health.* Instituto Centro Americano de la Salud, Managua, Nicaragua.

Mushi, A., J. Armstrong Schellenberg, H. Mponda, and C. Lengeler. "Targeted Subsidy for Malaria Control with Treated Nets Using a Discount Voucher System in Southern Tanzania." *Health Policy and Planning,* 18: 163-171.

Oberlander, J. 1998. "Remaking Medicare: The Voucher Myth." *Int J Health Serv* 281: 29–46.

O'Donnell, L.N., A. Sandoval, R. Duran and C. O'Donnell. 1995. "Video-Based Sexually Transmitted Disease Patient Education: Its Impact on Condom Acquisition." *American Journal of Public Health* 85: 817–822.

O'Neill, D.M 1977. "Voucher Funding of Training Programs: Evidence from the GI Bill." *Journal of Human Resources* 124: 425–45.

Patrinos, H., and D. Ariasingam 1997. *Decentralization of Education: Demand-Side Financing.* World Bank, Washington, DC.

Robey, B. 1987. "Community-Based Contraceptive Distribution: A Korean Success Story." *Asia-Pacific Population and Policy* 4: 1–4.

Roda, A. 2003. *Questionnaire for the World Bank Study on Voucher Schemes for Health.* Instituto Centro Americano de la Salud, Managua, Nicaragua.

Root, G. 2003. *Questionnaire for the World Bank Study on Voucher Schemes for Health.* Instituto CentroAmericano de la Salud, Managua, Nicaragua.

Sanderson, D., M. Place, and D. Wright. 2000. *Evaluation of the Powered Wheelchair and Voucher Scheme Initiatives.* York Health Economics Consortium, York: UK.

Sandiford, P., A. Gorter, and M. Salvetto. 2002a. "Use of Voucher Schemes for Output-Based Aid in the Health Sector in Nicaragua: Three Case Studies." Paper presented at the World Bank Workshop on Output-Based Aid, Frankfurt, January 24–26.

—. 2002b. "Vouchers for Health: Using Voucher Schemes for Output-Based Aid." *Public Policy for the Private Sector,* Viewpoint No. 243.

Sandiford P., M. Salvetto, Z. Segura, and A. Gorter 2000. "Clinics for Sex Workers in Managua." In *Public Services through Private Enterprise: Micro-Privatization for Improved Delivery,* ed. M. Harper. Pages 228-244. London: IT Publications.

Seidman, S.N., C. Sterk-Elifson, and S.O. Aral. 1994. "High-Risk Sexual Behavior among Drug-Using Men." *Sexually Transmitted Diseases,* May-June, 21(3): 173–180.

Silverman, K., M.A. Chutuape, G.E. Bigelow, and M.L. Stitzer. 1996. "Voucher-Based Reinforcement of Attendance by Unemployed Methadone Patients in a Job Skills Training Program." *Drug Alcohol Depend* 413: 197–207.

Simanowitz, A., B. Nkuna, and S. Kasim. 2000. "Overcoming the Obstacles of Identifying the Poorest Families: Using Participatory Wealth Ranking, the CASHPOR House Index, and Other Measurements to Identify and Encourage the Participation of the Poorest Families, Especially the Women of Those Families." Paper presented at the Microcredit Summit Meeting of Councils June 24–26.

Shaw, R.P. 1999. "New Trends in Public Sector Management in Health." Paper prepared for the World Bank Institute's Flagship on Health Sector Reform and Sustainable Financing, Washington, DC

Skaer, T.L., L.M. Robinson, D.A. Sclar, and G.H. Harding. 1996." Financial Incentive and the Use of Mammography among Hispanic Migrants to the United States." *Health Care Women Int* 174: 281–291.

Skibiak, J.P., M. Chambeshi-Moyo, and Y. Ahmed. 2001. *Testing Alternative Channels for Providing Emergency Contraception to Young Women. July.* Population Council, Washington, DC.

Slesinger, D.P., and C. Ofstead. 1996. "Using a Voucher System to Extend Health Services to Migrant Farm Workers." *Public Health Rep* 111(1): 57–62.

Sorensen, J.L., C.L. Masson, and A.L. Copeland. 1999. "Coupons/Vouchers as a Strategy for Increasing Treatment Entry for Opiate Dependent Injection Drug Users." In *Motivating Behavior Change among Illicit Drug Abusers: Contemporary Research on Contingency Management Interventions*, eds. S. Higgins and K. Silverman, 147–161. Washington, DC: American Psychological Association Press.

Steel, W. 2002. *Small Business Development Services: Kenya Voucher Program.* Seminar presented at the World Bank, Washington, DC. Presentation to Pro-poor Market Development Seminar, Series Social Capital Thematic Group by William F. Steel, Senior Adviser, Private Sector, Africa Region, World Bank, May 14, 2002.

Steuerle, E.C. 2000. "Common Issues for Voucher Programs." In *Vouchers and the Provision of Public Services*, eds. E.C. Steuerle, V.D. Ooms, G.E. Peterson, and R.D. Reishaver, 3–39. Washington, DC: Brookings Institution Press.

Stoner, T.J., B. Down, W.P. Carr, G. Maldonado, T.R. Church, and J. Mandel 1998. "Do Vouchers Improve Breast Cancer Screening Rates? Results from a Randomized Trial." *Health Serv Res* 331: 11–28.

Turner, S. 1997. "The Vision and Reality of Pell Grants: Unforeseen Consequences for Students and Institutions." Paper presented at the 25th Anniversary Pell Grant Conference, November 13–14, Washington DC.

U.S. Department of Justice and Federal Trade Commission. 1997. "Horizontal Merger Guidelines." Washington, DC. Available at http://www.usdoj.gov/atr/public/guidelines/horiz_book/toc.html.

Wagstaff, A., P. Paci, and E. Van Doorslaer. 1991. "On the Measurement of Inequalities in Health." *Social Science and Medicine* 33: 545–557.

Weinrich, S., D. Holdford, M. Boyd, D. Creanga, K. Cover, A. Johnson, M. Frank-Stromborg, and M. Weinrich. 1998. "Prostate Cancer Education in African American Churches." *Public Health Nursing* 15 (3): 188–95.

Weinrich, S.P., M.C. Weinrich, J. Priest, and C. Fodi. 2003. "Self-Reported Reasons

Men Decide Not to Participate in Free Prostate Cancer Screening." *Oncology Nursing Forum* 301: E12–E16.

West, Edwin G. 1996. "Education Vouchers in Practice and Principle: A World Survey." HCO Working Paper 64, World Bank, Human Capital Development and Operations Policy, Washington, DC.

Wortman, P.M., and R.G. St. Pierre. 1997. "The Educational Voucher Demonstration: A Secondary Analysis." *Education and Urban Society* 9(4): 471–92.

World Bank. No date. Reading List for Incidence Analysis: Poverty Impact Analysis. Washington, DC.

—. 1995. *Investing in People: The World Bank in Action.* Washington, DC: World Bank.

—. 2000. *Indonesia: Evaluating A Pilot Pro-Poor Safe Motherhood Project.* Poverty Net Library. Available at http//:www.poverty.worldbank.org/library/.

INDEX

A

abuse of voucher schemes, 37–38, 71
acceptance, 78
access rights, 76
adjudication, 80
administration, 20
adverse selection, 96
   monitoring for, 95
agency role, lack of institutional
      capacity, 40
appendices, 80
arbitration, 80

B

benefit incidence analysis, 98–99
benefit policies
   determining, 54–56, 57
   examples, 55
   limits, 57
benefits vs obstacles, 42
black markets, monitoring for, 94

C

capacity, lack of, 38
capitated payments, 6, 9, 12
cases, tracking and follow-up, 71
cash
   refunds, 8–9
   subsidies, 6
   transfers, 8
cervical cancer screening
   limits, 57
   prefeasibility assessment, 31–32
   provider selection, 62
   voucher design, 65

checklists
   feasibility assessment, 42
   prefeasibility assessment, 31
   voucher design, 72
cherry-picking. *See* cream-skimming
client satisfaction, 21
clinical records, 69
collusion, monitoring for, 93–94
communications, 66, 67, 78
   lack of, 40
competition, between providers, 13–15, 39,
      91–92
   absence of, 13–14
competitive voucher schemes, 17–21
context in which subsidies will be intro-
      duced, 29
contracting, 15, 77
contractors' responsibilities, 80
contracts
   elements, 78–80
   negotiating, 74–76
   tips, 75
contributions, 8
corruption, 15
cost-effectiveness, 4
   monitoring and evaluation, 100
cost-per-case contracts, 9
costs, 4, 5
   administrative, 12, 40
   fixed or predictable, 20–21
   transaction, 40
   voucher-bearer-borne, 57
counterfeiting
   monitoring for, 93
   prevention, 63–64
cream-skimming, 12
   monitoring for, 95–96